Digital Subtraction Imaging in Infants and Children

Edited by

Eric N. Faerber M.B., B.Ch., DMRD

Attending Radiologist
St. Christopher's Hospital for Children;
Associate Professor of Radiology
Temple University School of Medicine;
Clinical Associate Professor of Radiology
Medical College of Pennsylvania
School of Medicine,
and Hahnemann University School of Medicine
Philadelphia, Pennsylvania

1989
Futura Publishing Company, Inc.
Mount Kisco, New York

Library of Congress Cataloging-in-Publication Data

Digital subtraction imaging in infants and children/edited by Eric N. Faerber.

p. cm.

Includes index.

ISBN 0-87993-340-2

1. Digital subtraction angiography. 2. Pediatric cardiology.
I. Faerber, Eric N.

[DNLM: 1. Angiography—in infancy & childhood. 2. Subtraction Technic—in infancy & childhood. WG 500 D5745]

RJ423.5.D54D54 1988

618.92'1307572—dc 19

DNLM/DLC

for Library of Congress 88-24557

CIP

Published by

Futura Publishing Company, Inc.

295 Main Street, P.O. Box 330

Mount Kisco, New York 10549

L.C. no.: 88-24557

ISBN no.: 0-87993-340-2

Printed in the United States of America.

TO:

Marie A. Capitanio, M.D.
Alice Ettinger, M.D.
John C. Leonidas, M.D.
George L. Popky, M.D.
Samuel M. Wolpert, M.D.

A teacher affects eternity; he never knows where his influence stops.

Henry Brooks Adams (1838–1918)

Contributors

Suzanne E. Brickley, CCPT

Supervisor, Cardiovascular Laboratory, Department of Cardiology, St. Christopher's Hospital for Children, Philadelphia, Pennsylvania.

Marie A. Capitanio, M.D.

Director of Radiology, St. Christopher's Hospital for Children; Professor of Radiology, Temple University School of Medicine; Clinical Professor of Radiology, Medical College of Pennsylvania Hospital; Clinical Professor of Radiology, Hahnemann University School of Medicine, Philadelphia, Pennsylvania.

Kenneth S. Crystal, M.D.

Radiologist, Department of Radiology, New York Hospital; Assistant Professor of Radiology, Cornell University College of Medicine, New York, New York.

Richard M. Donner, M.D.

Chief of Cardiology, St. Christopher's Hospital for Children; Associate Professor of Cardiology and Pediatrics, Temple University School of Medicine, Philadelphia, Pennsylvania.

Eric N. Faerber, M.B., B.Ch., DMRD

Chief, Sections of Neuroradiology, Computed Tomography and Magnetic Resonance Imaging, St. Christopher's Hospital for Children; Associate Professor of Radiology, Temple University School of Medicine; Clinical Associate Professor of Radiology, Medical College of Pennsylvania School of Medicine; Clinical Associate Professor of Radiology, Hahnemann University School of Medicine, Philadelphia, Pennsylvania.

H. Theodore Harcke, M.D.

Director of Medical Imaging, Alfred I. Dupont Institute, Wilmington, Delaware; Clinical Associate Professor of Radiology and Pediatrics, Temple University School of Medicine; Clinical Associate Professor of Radiology (Pediatrics), Medical College of Pennsylvania, Philadelphia, Pennsylvania.

John A. Kirkpatrick, Jr., M.D.

Radiologist-In-Chief, Children's Hospital; Professor of Radiology, Harvard University School of Medicine, Boston, Massachusetts.

Calvin D. Neithamer, Jr., M.D.

Radiologist, Department of Radiology, New York Hospital; Assistant Professor of Radiology, Cornell University College of Medicine, New York, New York.

James N. Rauch, RCPT

Department of Cardiology, St. Christopher's Hospital for Children, Philadelphia, Pennsylvania.

Grigory Rozenblit, M.D.

Radiologist, Department of Radiology, New York Hospital; Assistant Professor of Radiology, Cornell University College of Medicine, New York, New York.

Eleanor Maloney Smergel, M.D.

Chief, Section of Angiography, St. Christopher's Hospital for Children; Assistant Professor of Radiology, Temple University School of Medicine; Clinical Assistant Professor, Medical College of Pennsylvania School of Medicine; Clinical Assistant Professor of Radiology, Hahnemann University School of Medicine, Philadelphia, Pennsylvania.

Thomas A. Sos, M.D.

Head, Division of Interventional and Cardiovascular Radiology, New York Hospital; Professor of Radiology, Cornell University College of Medicine, New York, New York.

Philip Stanley, M.D.

Head, Division of Diagnostic Radiology, Children's Hospital of Los Angeles; Professor of Radiology, University of Southern California School of Medicine, Los Angeles, California.

Ina L. D. Tonkin, M.D.

Professor of Radiology and Pediatrics, Department of Radiology, Le Bonheur Children's Medical Center, Memphis, Tennessee.

Arina van Breda, M.D.

Attending Radiologist, The Alexandria Hospital, Alexandria, Virginia; Assistant Clinical Professor of Radiology, George Washington University Medical Center, Washington, D.C.

Theodore Villafana, Ph.D.

Professor; Head, Diagnostic Physics, Temple University School of Medicine and Hospital, Philadelphia, Pennsylvania.

FOREWORD

The essence of this book is the imminence of our radiologic future. The authors, under the direction of Dr. Faerber, have demonstrated that all of radiology is immersed at the present in the practical application of digital techniques except those studies represented by plain films and for these, working prototypes are already in place in many departments. In order to understand the rapid strides that have been made in the digital production of images, the first chapter details the basic principles of digital subtraction angiography and the language of analog to digital conversion. Much that appears in this chapter is applicable to an understanding of digital techniques for imaging in general.

The following two chapters and the appendix are concerned not only with techniques but also with the design of appropriate housing for the units and finally with the application of the method to clinical angiography. All is not positive; in Chapter 3, it is noted that: "Whereas intravenous digital subtraction angiography was heralded as an effective replacement for conventional catheter arteriography, it has not lived up to its early promise and is now reserved for special circumstances." At the same time, the advantages of intra-arterial digital subtraction angiography are noted, specifically the immediate availability of the image and the smaller volume of contrast material required for an image, factors of immediate importance to the examination of the infant and child.

This somewhat general approach to digital subtraction techniques for peripheral angiography is complemented by Chapter 4 which deals with digital angiocardiography and by Chapters 5–8 which deal with specific vessels and organs, i.e., the aorta, the cerebral and renal vessels, and *those* of the extremities. In some instances there is an overlap from one chapter to another but when that occurs it is apparent that the authors and the editor feel that the resulting emphasis is of importance.

Chapter 9 deals with future applications and trends in digital imaging and sets the stage for expectations in the near and not so near future. There is no question that uncomplicated storage and easy retrieval of data are hurdles to be overcome, but in the process of solving those problems, the problems of the present file room will be solved. Storage, retrieval, and display of the stored information and the design of a network, i.e., where should the links be with the system within the department of radiology and within the hospital. The conclusion of that chapter is concerned with the future and the author notes that the future is closer than we think. It is stated that perhaps twenty-five percent of the total examinations in some departments are in the digital format. These include, of course, computed tomography, nuclear medicine, ultrasonography, magnetic resonance imaging, and techniques for angiography and angiocardiography. In an increasing number of departments, there is ongoing research into the application of presently available digital radiography units.

These units have drawbacks, but they also are of such quality that their promise can readily be appreciated. However, not only must digital techniques pass the test of comparison with radiographs, they also require the education of clinicians and radiologists in their use, e.g., a different size and format. Perhaps we are not quite ready for "consensus" interpretation of studies performed in our departments but this will come just as surely as the computer terminal will replace the viewbox, as stated by the author of Chapter 9.

This book is an exciting look at a future that is very close to being the present and presents digital techniques, in use and promised, with all of their advantages and disadvantages for the consideration of the reader. In so doing, the text also presents a succinct review of a spectrum of pediatric disorders.

John A. Kirkpatrick, Jr., M.D.
Professor of Radiology
Harvard Medical School
Radiologist-in-Chief
Children's Hospital
Boston, Massachusetts

PREFACE

Digital subtraction imaging is yet another milestone in the relentless path of radiologic progress. Since the momentous discovery of x-rays by Wilhelm Roentgen in 1895, conventional radiography has been augmented by fluoroscopy, tomography, angiography, radionuclide scanning, ultrasonography, computed tomography, and magnetic resonance imaging.

Angiography dates back to December 1895 when Haschek in Vienna performed an angiogram on an amputated hand. Angiography has steadily progressed from the pioneering work of Egas Moniz in 1927 to the sophisticated angiographic techniques presently available. Intravenous angiography was performed in 1939 by Robb and Steinberg, but then was largely abandoned until the advent of electronic techniques devised in America and Germany in the 1970s.

The current role of digital imaging in both the pediatric and adult age groups is still evolving. There is considerable difference in technique as evidenced in the following chapters from the many distinguished authors. The aim of this monograph on digital subtraction angiography in infants and children is to provide information on the techniques available and the indications for this modality. The co-authors are pre-eminent in their respective fields and have already contributed greatly to the radiologic literature.

I am very grateful to the many people who have aided me in the preparation of this monograph. Marie Capitanio, M.D., has been the major source of help and inspiration. She has helped nurture this project, and has also considerably assisted in the editing of the manuscript. I am indebted to George Popky, M.D., for my initiation into digital subtraction angiography and for making many resources available to our patients. The Department of Cardiology at St. Christopher's Hospital for Children continues to be of great assistance to us. Therefore, I wish to gratefully acknowledge Drs. Iain Black, Richard Donner, Anna O'Riordan, Terry Anderson, Lloyd Marks, Giullermo Sanchez, Ashok Mehta, Craig Cohen, and David Burton; and also Suzanne Brickley, George Luks, James Rauch, and Victor Raspaldo.

The librarial assistance of Martha Kirby and Nancy Washburne Haines is also very much appreciated. It is again with much gratitude that I acknowledge the secretarial assistance of Joan Colombaro, who has painstakingly assisted me in the preparation of this monograph.

I am indebted to my publisher, Steven Korn, of Futura Publishing Company. He has been a major source of enthusiasm, assistance and good counsel throughout the preparation of this monograph. His patience and good sense of humor have been indispensable to me. I also have been fortunate to have the superb editorial assistance of Judith Bianciardi and Linda Shaw. It has been a great pleasure working with them.

My wife Esmè and children, Jennifer and Michael, have once again offered unlimited moral support and have made many sacrifices on my behalf.

Eric N. Faerber, M.B., B.Ch., DMRD

CONTENTS

Chapter 1

Basic Physics and Instrumentation for Digital Subtraction Angiography

THEODORE VILLAFANA

An understanding of the physical principles of digital subtraction angiography results in the more intelligent application of this imaging modality in clinical situations. Subtraction angiography has been performed by angiographers for many years using standard film screen cassette technology. Film subtraction techniques, however, have a number of disadvantages and limitations which are circumvented by the digital approach. The purpose of this chapter is twofold: (1) to briefly review the process of film subtraction as well as its limitations; and (2) to present the principles and the advantages of digital subtraction techniques.

Film Subtraction

Figure 1 illustrates structures that are clustered close to each other as well as superimposed upon each other. Clustering and superimposition interfere with the accurate localization and clear definition of a structure of interest on a radiograph. Subtle image features and deviations from normal are difficult to detect when structures are clustered and superimposed. When one structure lies above another structure on a radiograph of a patient, the structure that is most dense will dominate the gray scale and make radiographic visualization of the other structure difficult. The subtraction process provides for the elimination of those structures in an image which are not germane to the examination.

Digital Subtraction Imaging in Infants and Children, edited by Eric N. Faerber. Mount Kisco, New York: Futura Publishing Company, Inc., © 1989.

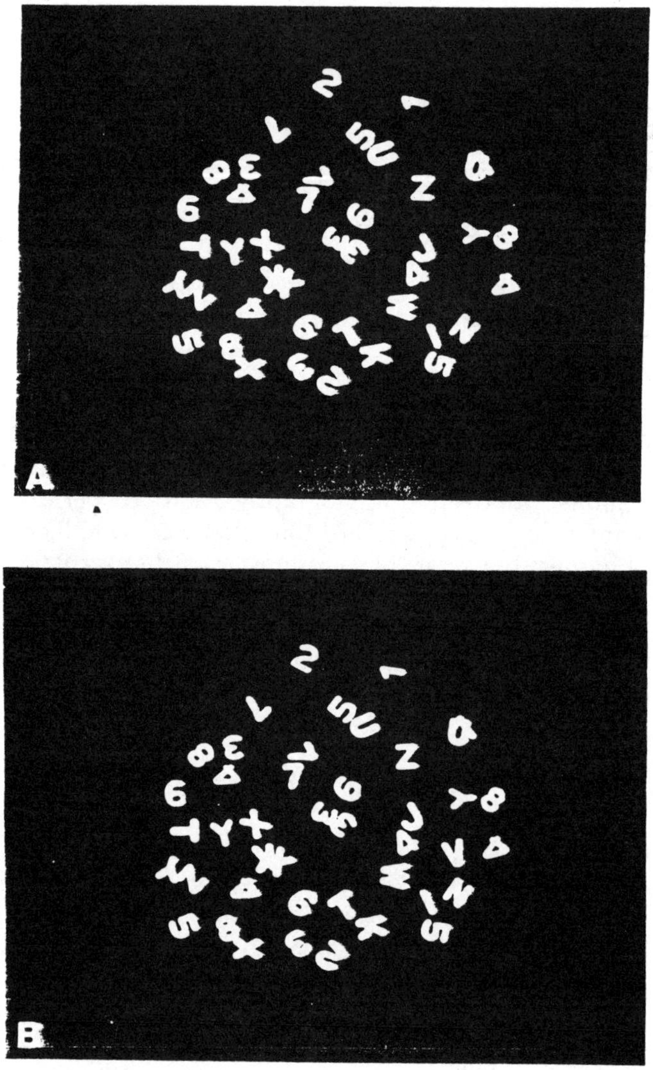

*FIGURE 1. Clustering and superimposition. Visualization of detail is greatly diminished in the presence of clustering and superimposition of features. Note the letter V in (**B**) but not in (**A**); when (**A**) is subtracted from (**B**) only the letter V remains (**C**).*

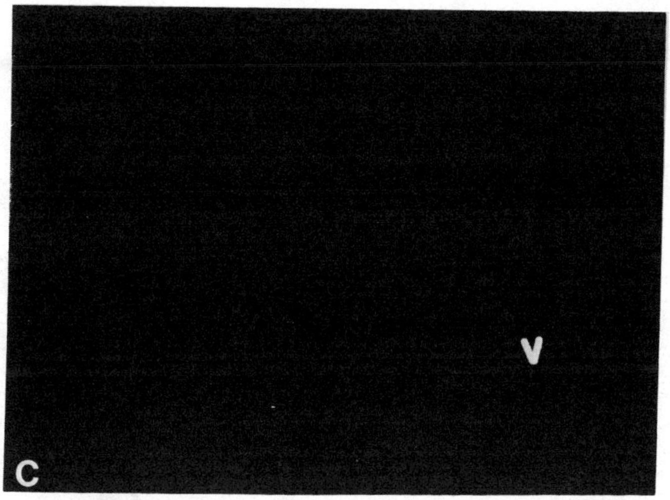

Figure 1C.

The Film Subtraction Process

Two radiographs of the part are essential to perform the subtraction process. The first radiograph or scout film of the anatomic region of interest will contain all of the anatomic information that will subsequently be subtracted out. To accomplish the subtraction, the grey scale present on the scout film is inverted by placing the scout film in contact with a special, commercially available subtraction film and then passing light through both of them. After processing the subtraction film, the net result is the original image with all its densities inverted. This inverted image is referred to as the mask image. (Fig. 2) When the scout and the mask images are sandwiched together, each area on the scout film overlaps its inverted image on the mask film so that an area that is black overlaps an area that is white. If the two films are then placed in contact with a third film and light passed through them, the net density at every point of the resulting image will be an overall, intermediate, uniform gray density. All the information recorded on the original scout film is eliminated (Fig. 3). Thus, to obtain the final subtracted image, additional radiographs of the same anatomic region are obtained, but with the injection of contrast media into the vessels of interest. The resulting image is referred to as the live image because information is present that was not present in the original scout film. If the mask image is combined with the live image and the subtraction process carried out as described above, all of the information on the live image that was present on the mask image (background tissue structures) will be subtracted out. The only information remaining on the final image will be the opacified vessels. This simple film subtraction technique provides for a significant increase in the visualization of vascular structures, which is essential for accurate diagnosis in angiography.

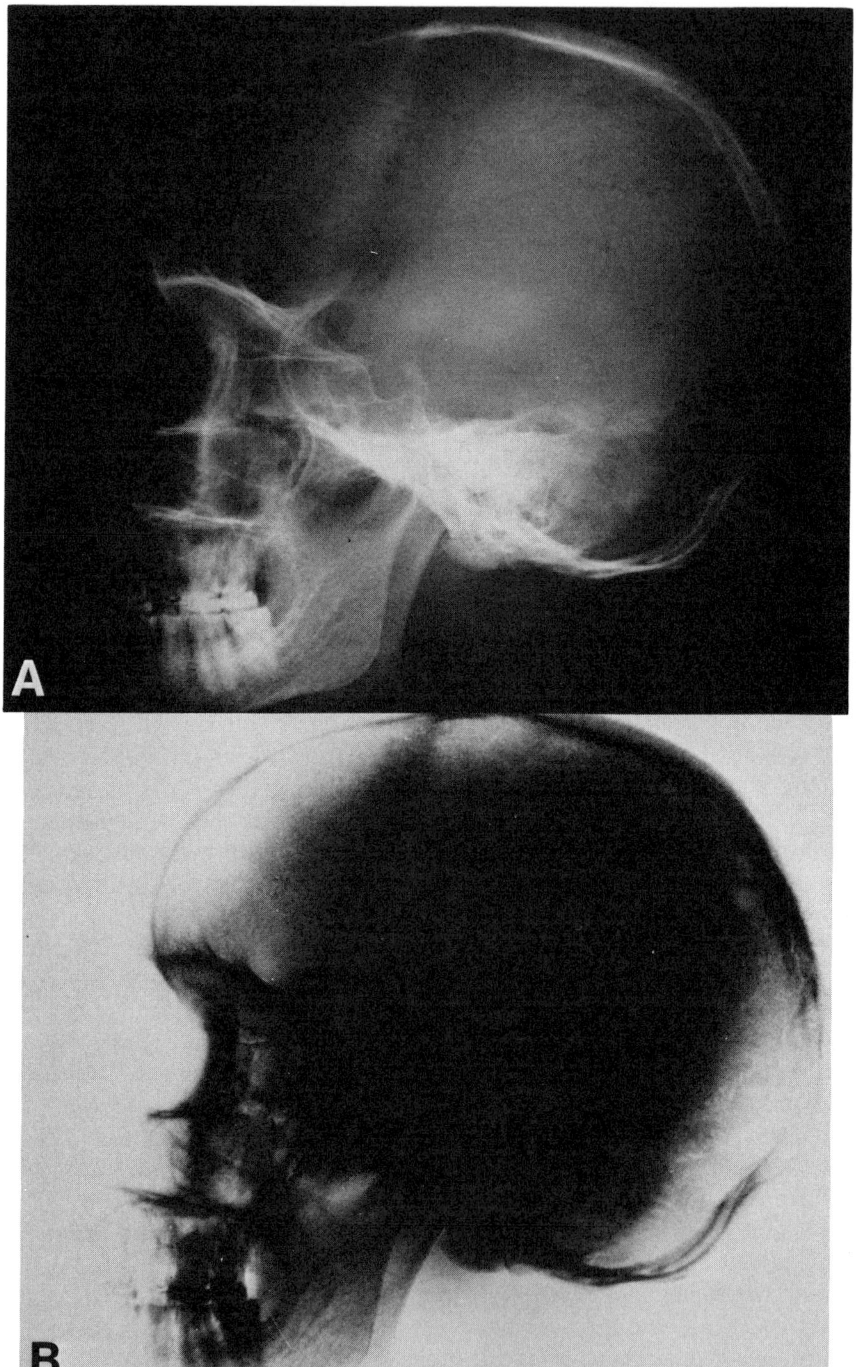

*FIGURE 2. Scout and mask images. The mask image (**B**) is identical to the scout image (**A**) except that the gray scale has been inverted. The dark areas on the scout image appear as light areas on the mask image. If these two images were to be superimposed one on the other, then each dark area would cancel each corresponding light area resulting in a "blank image."*

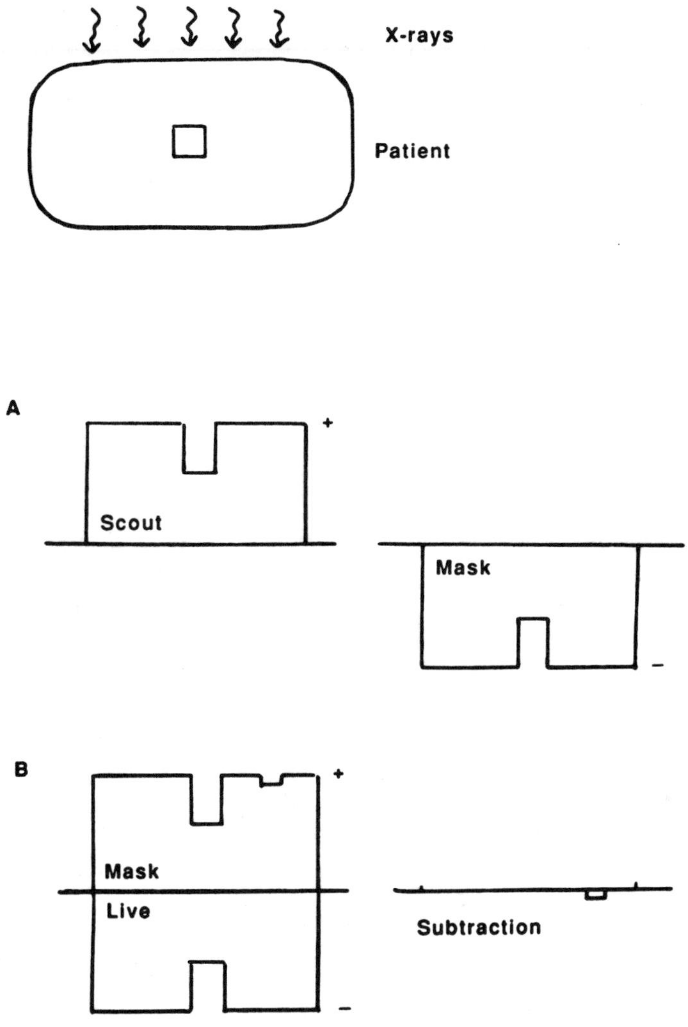

FIGURE 3. Image profile drawings obtained from a given cross section of a hypothetical patient as x-rays penetrate through to the detector. **A**: *X-ray intensity distribution emerging from a hypothetical patient with just one image feature present, a square absorbing tissue block. This results in a density distribution on the scout film; the mask image shows the inverted gray scale.* **B**: *If the mask image with the gray scale inverted is combined with a live image containing a contrast-filled blood vessel in addition to the original background features, then a uniform gray image results which is devoid of all background features and shows only the image of the blood vessel.*

As noted above, the superimposition effect leads to the possibility of one structure dominating the gray scale, thereby reducing the available latitude. An added feature of the subtraction process is that latitude is greatly enhanced. Thus, a greater range of image features can be displayed with more optimal densities by use of subtraction techniques (Fig. 4).

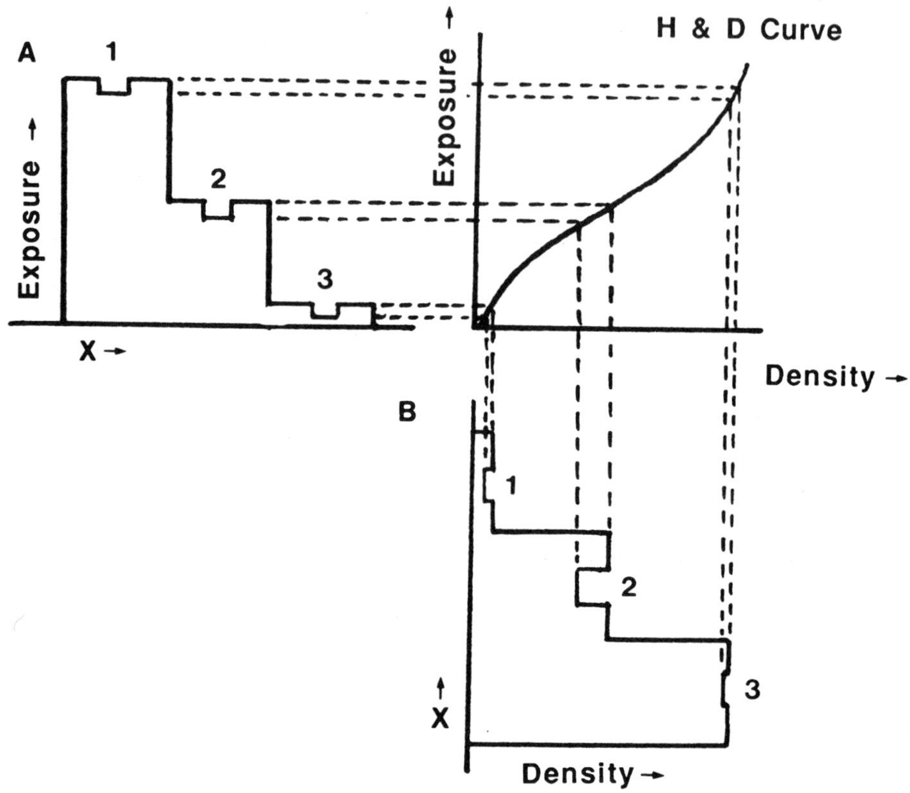

FIGURE 4. *Expansion of the available image latitude by the film subtraction process.* **A**: *Exposure pattern emerging from the patient.* **B**: *The final density pattern recorded is dependent on the particular H & D curve characteristic used. Vessels #1 and #3, having high and low x-ray transmission in the surrounding tissues, respectively, would fall in the overexposed and underexposed regions of the H & D curve where image contrast is limited. Vessel #2, however, falls in the middle of the available density region and is optimally visualized because of the greater resulting density differences. After subtraction, all three vessels are displayed independent of surrounding tissues.*

Limitation of Film Subtraction Angiography

The primary limitation is the interval of time that transpires between obtaining the scout, mask, and live images, when the patient is apt to move. If the patient moves, the live image will not be spatially oriented exactly as the scout image. Consequently, structures will not subtract out exactly since their borders will not line up exactly. This is referred to as a misregistration.

A somewhat similar limitation to the film subtraction process is that the live image is manually aligned or registered with the mask image. In order to obtain a successful subtraction, the alignment must be exact. Misaligning the images will produce the same results as does patient motion (Figs. 5 and 6).

Another limitation relates to the fact that radiographic film is notoriously

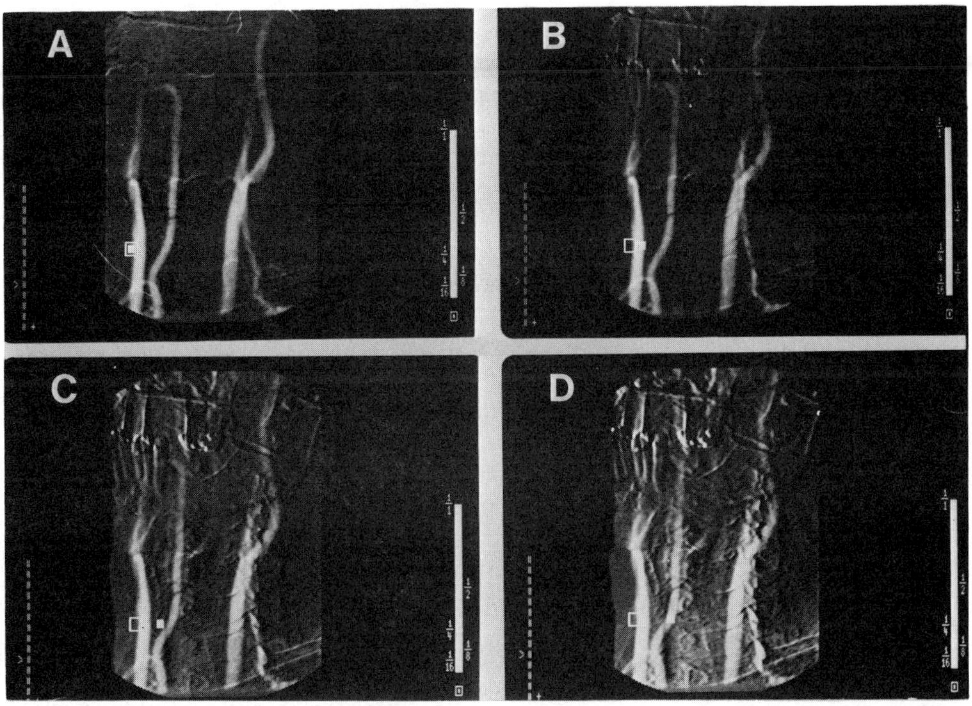

FIGURE 5. Misregistration. **A**: *Image is in register (no motion).* **B–D**: *Images are misregistered by 1-, 2- and 3-pixel dimensions, respectively. Note that each misregistered border is characterized by an adjacent dark and light area and that image visualization is greatly degraded. These digitally produced images were misregistered by digitally shifting the mask and live images (pixel shifting).*

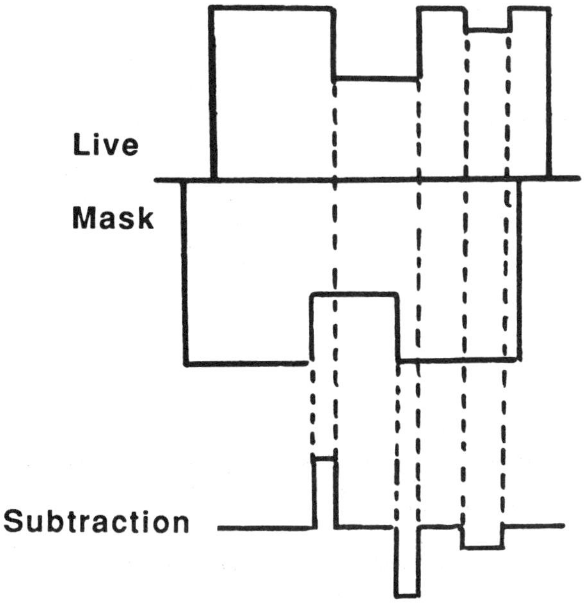

FIGURE 6. Misregistration Artifact. Image profiles illustrating the theoretical basis of the misregistration artifact. When the live image is shifted relative to the mask image, the borders do not line up and the resulting subtracted image has features with both black and white borders.

nonlinear. Therefore, exact inversion is not totally possible since the high-density shoulder area does not coincide exactly with the low-density toe area.

Lastly, tedious manual labor is necessary to perform the film subtraction process. More often than not, therefore, fewer images are subtracted than would be the case if a less time-consuming process were available.

Digital Subtraction Instrumentation

The physical principles involved in digital subtraction angiography (DSA) are similar to those involved in film subtraction angiography. The difference, however, lies in the manner in which the images are acquired and the subtraction process carried out. In the case of DSA, the images are acquired via fluoroscopy and converted into a digital form. The digital images are then transmitted directly to a digital computer where the appropriate mask images are subtracted digitally from subsequent live images. The computer is an ideal instrument to perform the necessary repetitive subtraction steps. The advanced digital systems even provide for a real-time display (30 frames/sec) of the final subtracted images. Interested readers are referred to the literature for an historical account of DSA.[1]

A diagram of a complete digital subtraction angiography system is illustrated in Figure 7. In the digitial subtraction system, the x-rays passing through the patient are detected by an image intensifier arrangement typically used in fluoroscopy. The image intensifier intensifies the image and, utilizing an optical

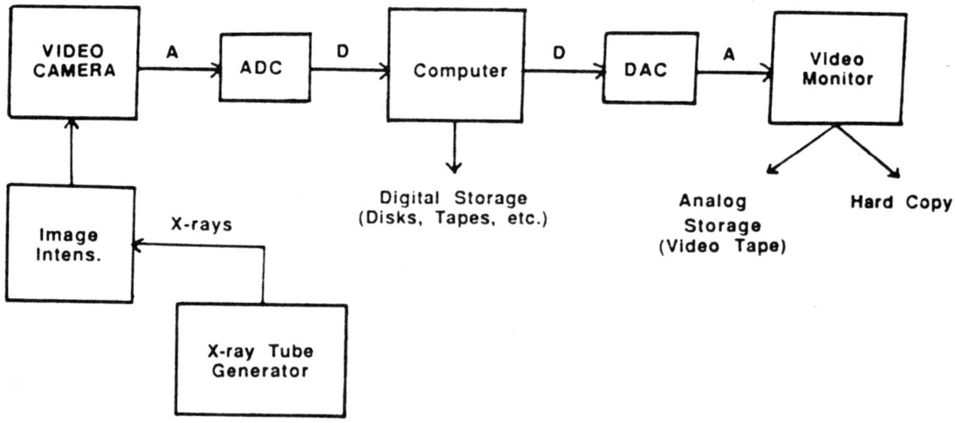

FIGURE 7. Block diagram of a typical DSA system. X-rays emerging from the patient are converted to light in the image intensifier and detected with the video camera. Output signal from camera is in analog form (A) and is converted to digital form (D) at the analog-to-digital converter (ADC). After processing in the computer, the data in digital form (D) is converted back to analog form (A) at the digital-to-analog converter (DAC). The image is now suitable for video viewing.

system, the image is viewed by a video camera which then passes the image to the computer for manipulation and storage. Since the signal from the video camera is a continuous voltage signal and thus in analog form, it must be converted to digital form. This is done by a device known as the analog-to-digital converter (ADC).

The type of video camera used in nondigital fluoroscopy is the Vidicon, whereas the camera used in the digital approach is the Plumbicon. Although the two types of video cameras are similar, the Plumbicon provides for enhanced spatial and temporal resolution as well as enhanced sensitivity characteristics. After the digital subtraction image is produced, it must be displayed at the video monitor which is an analog device. The digital data are converted back to analog form by the digital-to-analog converter (DAC). A copy of the video displayed image may be obtained using the multiformat camera and stored for future reference. We will now look in depth into each component of this chain.

The Generator and the X-Ray Tube

The important parameters associated with the x-ray tube and generator are interdependent. The generator supplies the high voltage (kV peak) and the x-ray tube current. The higher the kVp the greater the photon penetration through the patient. Most generator systems are capable of supplying up to 150 kVp. The levels needed for DSA are typically between 75 and 115 kVp. The x-ray tube current, measured in milliamperes (mA), is determined by the number of electrons being accelerated between the filament and the anode target within the x-ray tube. The combination of kVp, mA and exposure time is referred to as the heat load. Each x-ray tube has a certain heat load capacity which must not be exceeded.

To perform DSA, short time intervals are usually necessary in order to avoid patient or vessel motion during the exposure and to allow high framing rates. To achieve short exposure intervals, between 1,000 and 2,000 mA are necessary. An important consideration is the capability of the x-ray focal spot to withstand such high, instantaneous heat loads. It is to no avail to configure a system with a generator of high output capability and an x-ray tube of low heat capacity. This is especially critical when a small focal spot is required for enhanced resolution and for magnification studies. When a small focal spot is used, the heat energy concentration is over a small region and may result in exceeding the heat capacity of the tube and subsequent damage to the tube. The heat load expressed in heat units (HU) for a particular DSA run is defined as the product of the number of images (N) in that run, the peak kilovoltage as kVp, the tube current (mA), and the exposure time for each image in seconds or $HU = 1.35\ N \times kVp \times mA \times sec$. The factor 1.35 is a constant that takes into account the fact that DSA systems typically use three-phase generators.

Every x-ray tube has a heat unit capacity which the focal spot cannot exceed; if exceeded it results in a target melt down or other damage to the tube. The x-ray tubes used in typical DSA systems have heat unit capacities in the order of 500,000 to 1,000,000 HU. This is significantly greater than that of tubes used in routine radiography which have heat unit capacities in the order of 75,000 to 200,000 HU.

The greater the heat capacity of the tube, the smaller the focal spots that can be utilized. This is of particular importance for magnification techniques since image unsharpness due to the size of the focal spot is also magnified. The size of the focal spot used in DSA should, as a rule, not exceed 1.3 mm.

A tube with a high heat capacity allows for a greater framing rate which is an important consideration in angiography. In DSA a maximum of 4 or 5 images/sec are usually sufficient; however, in angiocardiography as many as 30 images/sec may be required.

The tube heat capacity also has an effect on the image matrix size. Large matrix sizes imply smaller pixel sizes and thus greater spatial resolution. Smaller pixel sizes, in turn, imply fewer x-ray quanta per pixel and thus greater quantum mottle or x-ray noise generated. To avoid this, the input x-ray photon levels and the tube load must be increased. To be more specific, a doubling of the matrix size from 512 × 512 to 1024 × 1024 implies a fourfold increase in the number of pixels and a doubling of the potential spatial resolution available along any direction in the image. However, since this results in a fourfold decrease in the number of photons available for each pixel, a fourfold increase in the x-ray output is required to maintain the same x-ray noise characteristics.

Another consideration is whether the generator allows for rapid kVp switching which is required for dual-energy imaging. Dual-energy techniques are still in the experimental stages, although their potential is well recognized.[1,2]

The Image Intensifier

The internal components of an image intensifier are illustrated in Figure 8. The x-rays that emerge from the patient impinge on the input phosphor where the x-ray energy is absorbed and converted to light. Modern day input phosphors are made of cesium iodide (CsI). The light emitted from the input phosphor falls upon a second layer, the photocathode, resulting in the emission of electrons. The electrons emitted from the photocathode are then accelerated by a voltage difference across the image intensifier towards another phosphor layer called the output phosphor. During acceleration, a series of electrostatic focusing lenses focus the electrons onto the relatively small output phosphor. When the electrons fall upon the output phosphor visible light is once again emitted. The emitted light, however, is now greatly intensified and is gathered and projected forward by the objective lens. The light image at this point is ready to be detected by an appropriate image pickup device such as a video camera, a 105-mm film camera, or a cine camera.

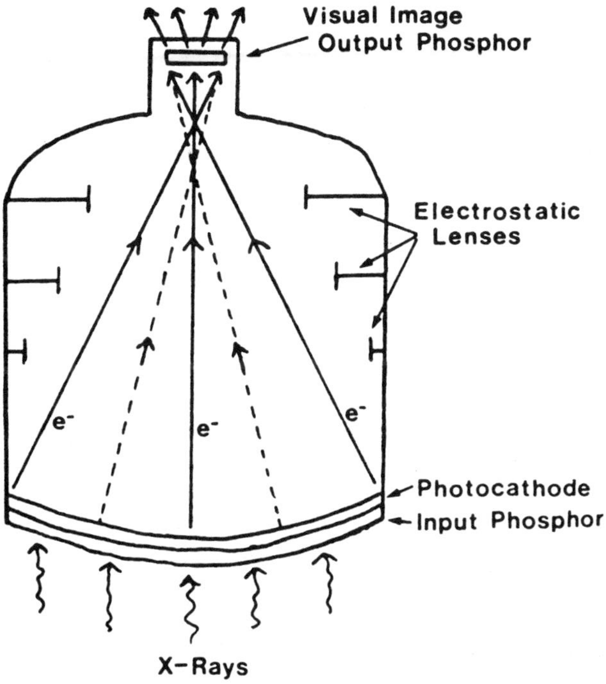

FIGURE 8. Internal components of an image intensifier tube. X-rays are converted to light at the input phosphor. The light image is then converted to an electron distribution at the photocathode. These electrons are accelerated across the tube and focused via electrostatic lenses onto smaller output phosphors where the final visual light image emerges. In order to accomplish image intensified magnification, a smaller region of the input phosphor is chosen via the electrostatic focusing lenses to occupy the full size of the output phosphor (dashed lines). The net result is that smaller features appear larger at the monitor.

Dual-Field Fluoroscopy

Image magnification is possible with an image intensifier without the need to change the geometry of the patient and the x-ray tube as is necessary in radiography. If there is a small structure at the input phosphor to be visualized, the electrons can be picked off over a smaller region of the input phosphor (Fig. 8). This is accomplished by adjusting the bias on the electrostatic lenses, such that only electrons emerging from the desired area on the photocathode are focused at the output phosphor. This has the net effect of mapping a smaller area of the photocathode onto the full output phosphor and thus magnifying the image finally viewed at the video monitor. In addition to dual mode, trifield image intensifiers are available in which there are three different fields from which to choose. Each smaller field yields a greater degree of magnification. Typical field combinations are 12, 9, and 6 in or 9, 6, and 4½ in. The greater the degree of magnification, the greater the radiation dose to the patient.

Video Cameras

The light that emerges from the output phosphor diverges in all directions. The objective lens efficiently gathers and projects the light forward in a manner suitable for detection by an appropriate pickup device such as a video camera.

Video cameras are of two generic classes: Vidicons and Orthicons. The typical configuration of a Vidicon camera is illustrated in Figure 9. Vidicons are relatively small, rugged, and cheap to manufacture. The Orthicon type cameras have the advantage of greater spatial and temporal resolution, as well as greater sensitivity. However, Orthicons are more complex, larger, fragile, and more expensive. As a consequence, Orthicons are not used routinely in fluoroscopy or in DSA systems. Since DSA requires a higher performance camera than the Vidicon, a Plumbicon camera is utilized. A Plumbicon camera is essentially a Vidicon; however, its target plate is made of a special lead monoxide layer. Such a configuration allows the Plumbicon to have better spatial resolution and sensitivity properties compared to the standard Vidicon.

In forming the image, the electron gun scans the target plate in a series of so-called raster lines. These lines, as well as the number of image signal samples obtained along the scan line, determine the maximum resolution performance of the system. Typically, both broadcast video and conventional fluoroscopy use 525-raster line systems. If greater resolution is desired cameras capable of scanning greater number of lines such as 1,000 lines would then be necessary.

There are two ways of reading out the video camera target plate: (1) to use an interlace pattern and (2) to use a progressive, consecutive line-by-line approach. The interlace approach is the conventional one utilized in 525-line fluoroscopy and broadcast video. Interlaced readout consists of the electron gun

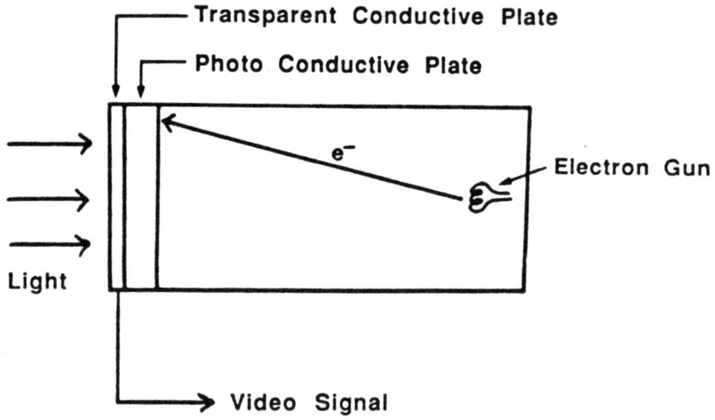

FIGURE 9. Diagram of a Vidicon camera. Incident light passes through a transparent conductive plate on to a photoconductive target plate. Simultaneously the electrons from the electron gun are accelerated in a fine beam and fall on the target plate. The electronic current across this plate depends on the photoconductivity produced by the incident light at each point. The resulting current, which is proportional to the light at each point, is conducted by the conductive plate and constitutes the video signal.

making two scans over the full target (Fig. 9). The first pass picks up half of the 525 lines over the full screen and the second pass picks up every other line in interlace fashion. Although adequate for continuous mode fluoroscopy, its use has serious drawbacks in DSA which is implemented with a series of x-ray pulses. In the pulsed DSA progressive readout approach, each line is read out sequentially. This approach more effectively uses the full number of lines available at the camera target plate with a resulting increase in signal-to-noise ratio. In addition, the progressive readout approach results in significant radiation dose savings.

No matter which readout approach is utilized, the analog signal from the video camera is digitized at the ADC and then passed to the computer where the proper computations are performed. Because video monitors are analog devices, the signal from the computer is transformed back to analog form by the digital-to-analog converter (DAC) before the image can be displayed.

Analog-to-Digital Converter (ADC)

For the computer to perform the proper computations, the video signal must be digitized (Fig. 10). This is the function of the ADC. The analog signal must be digitized both in space and intensity. Spatial digitization consists of dividing the spatial dimensions into a matrix array of individual pixels (*pi*cture *el*ements). Typical arrays in DSA fall between 256 by 256 to 512 by 512. More recent state of the art units have matrix arrays as large as 1024 by 1024. Note that for any

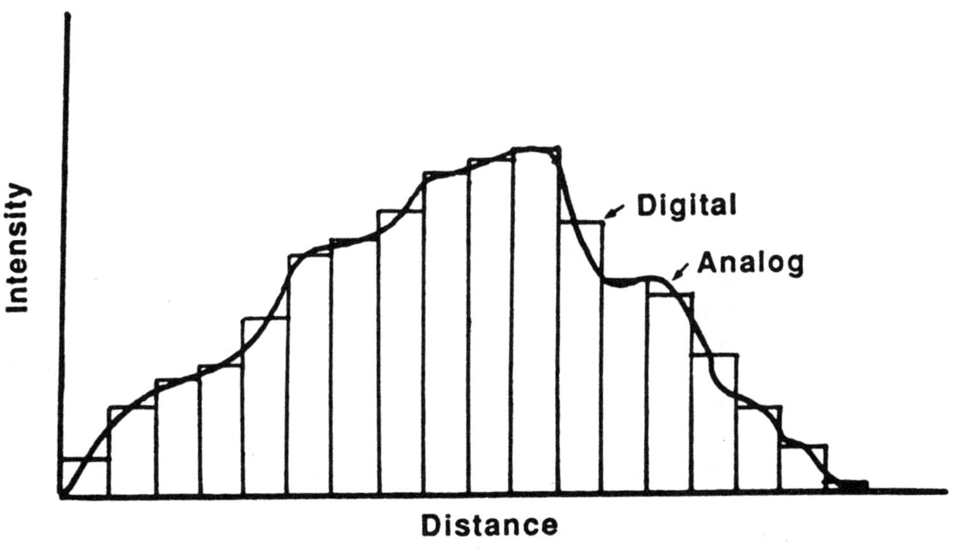

FIGURE 10. Conversion of an analog video signal to a digital signal. Both distance and image intensity must be digitized as shown in the histogram above. The distance is digitized into a pixel array. The digitization of the image intensity is referred to as the bit depth.

one pixel, a value for the intensity is chosen by providing for a discrete number of intensity levels. This defines the final gray scale that will be available. It is conventional to describe the gray scale in bits expressed in powers of two. Thus 4 gray levels is given by 2^2 or 2 bits. A bit is the fundamental unit of information for the computer and can assume one of two values, zero or one. For example, a complete digitization of an image may be designated as $256 \times 256 \times 8$. This means that there are 256×256 pixels and that each pixel is divided into 2^8 or 256 gray levels. The number of gray levels is also referred to as the bit depth. Thus 256 gray levels are also referred to as an 8-bit image.

In general, the greater the matrix size and number of gray levels, the greater the potential image quality. First, quantum mottle rises since an increase in the number of pixels results in fewer x-ray photons available per pixel. Therefore as an image is divided into small parts, the number of x-ray photons contributing to any pixel is less. To overcome the problem of noise, the radiation dose to the patient may have to be increased. Second, the number of frame rates may have to be reduced, since a greater matrix size and/or gray level size implies that more data need to be processed leading to an overall reduction in throughput time. To overcome this problem, more costly, higher capacity/greater memory computer systems, would be necessary. Finally, storage capacity would be diminished, since greater matrix size and/or gray level scale imply that more data must be stored. Again, this would demand additional, higher storage capacity devices and associated higher costs to solve the problem.

Computer

Once the video signal is digitized, the subtraction process is performed by the computer. There are relatively large variations in the types of computers used in DSA. In all cases the computer has two main purposes. One purpose or function is system control. For instance, the computer can control the image acquisition function, generation of the x-ray generator, and the exposure factor settings. The other function of the computer is to perform mathematical and logical operations on the image data as well as to carry out image processing. There is a strong trend to distribute the functions of the computer by having smaller microprocessor units at various points in the system performing specific functions. This aids in speeding up the overall processing time and allows for the simultaneous performance of separate tasks. The internal configuration of the computer also provides for random access memory (RAM) which is usually configured into three frames. Each frame is capable of holding full-image data. Two memory frames hold image data that are just acquired (Fig. 11). Mathematical manipulations of the image data, such as subtraction, are performed within the arithmetic logic unit (ALU) of the computer and the results are stored in the display memory. The data in the display memory are subsequently transferred to hard disk, short-term storage and are available for viewing at the video monitor.

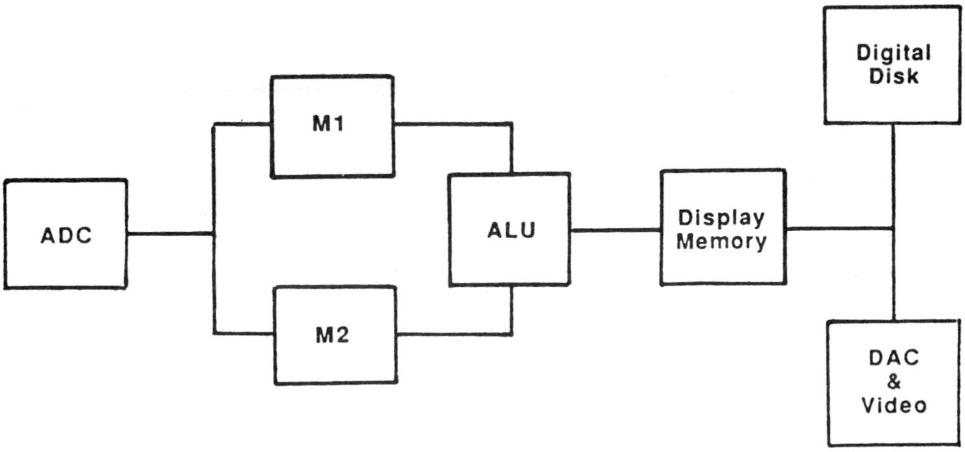

FIGURE 11. *Typical configuration of a modern DSA computer system. Digital information is fed into two memory frames (M1 and M2). The arithmetic logic unit (ALU) performs the mathematical manipulation between two images and the result is stored in the display memory. The image is subsequently transferred to hard disk storage in digital form and is also available at the video monitor in analog form for viewing.*

Video Monitor and Hard Copy Devices

As noted, provision must be made to display the digital image. One device to display the image is a video monitor in which case the line capacity of the monitor must be taken into consideration. If the original image was 512 × 512, then the typical 525-line video systems would be adequate. High-resolution video monitors having 1,000 lines could yield greater image quality. However, such monitors should be matched to video cameras that have an output of 1,000 lines for optimal results. In order to achieve very high-resolution capacity, the data that are to be processed should be collected in a digital array of 1024 × 1024 and with greater bit depths.

For optimal gray scale control at the video monitor, windowing can be performed in a manner similar to that performed in viewing computerized tomographic imaging. This is necessary, since the dynamic range of the system is sufficiently large that all of the data cannot be displayed at any one time on the available gray scale of the video display. Windowing makes it possible to choose a subset of the data and display only that data using the given brightness range of the video monitor.

Lastly, a final hard copy may be produced by using a multiformat camera. The multiformat camera consists of an additional independent video monitor from which images are flashed onto a film for permanent recording. Recently, laser imagers have been introduced. These have the potential for greater resolution and contrast properties because the video monitor is totally bypassed and the image signal from the DAC directly modulates the intensity of the laser beam that is scanning across a film. Future versions of the laser scanner promise to record the digital image information directly from the computer bypassing the digital to analog device and its associated image degradation.

Image Storage

In addition to viewing the image at the video monitor, it is important that both short- and long-term storage of the image be available. There are a number of different types of storage devices available in DSA. These include digital disks, digital magnetic tapes, digital cartridges, floppy disks, and hard disks.

In general, the most important parameters to be considered are the storage capacity of the device and how quickly the images can be read in or off the device. For example, floppy disks are very convenient because they are relatively small, flexible, and easily stored. However, floppy disks have limited storage capacity and in some applications more than one disk is needed to record all of the images in the study of a single patient. Magnetic tape, on the other hand, has a very large storage capacity, but access time is relatively long since it is a serial access device. Images are recorded on magnetic tape serially, one after each other. Therefore, if the image desired is recorded near the end of the tape, it is necessary to proceed through all of the images to find the desired image. Similarly, if the desired image is at the beginning of the tape, it is necessary to rewind the tape and then to go through each image serially until the desired image is reached. The use of magnetic tapes is time consuming, cumbersome, and more importantly often impedes patient throughput. Although some modern tape recorders operate at high speed, have automatic threading, winding, and unwinding, the disadvantages noted above are lessened but not eliminated.

All DSA systems have Winchester hard disks for on-line, short-term storage. By virtue of these random access devices, images can be accessed directly and rapidly. In general, less than 1,000 images can be stored in these devices unless more disk platters are utilized which then increases the cost of the system. In addition to digital storage, analog storage devices such as video tape are also available. In video taping, the images are recorded directly off the video monitor. In general, digital storage devices are preferred to analog devices because digital-to-analog transformation results in some image degradation. Image degradation also occurs using video tape devices and the video monitor.

The laser or optical disk promises to revolutionize image storage. The laser disk operates in a manner similar to the Winchester disk, but the information is recorded differently. In the case of the Winchester disk, information is recorded on a magnetic recording medium. The recording of information using laser disks is accomplished by burning small, micron size holes into an appropriate medium by means of a laser beam. As a result, the amount of information that can be recorded is greatly increased because laser-produced holes can be packed very closely together. A single laser disk platter is capable of storing more than 50,000 images compared to the several hundred images that can be stored on a hard disk.

Image storage capacity is determined by the number of bits per digitized image. Storage capacity is usually specified in bytes and can be calculated as follows:

$$\text{Megabytes/image} = \frac{\text{Matrix size} \times \text{bit depth}}{8} + 1{,}024$$

There are 8 bits in a byte, thus the 8 in the denominator converts bits to bytes and 1,024 represents the number of bytes needed for the patient identification and image header information. For example a 256 × 256 × 10 image would need (256 × 256 × 10)/8 + 1024 = 82,944 bytes/image or 0.08MB/image. It is apparent that any increases in matrix size and/or bit depth will quickly increase the number of bytes needed to store an image.

When making decisions that affect image quality such as matrix size and bit depth (gray scale digitization), these decisions will directly affect the computer capacity and image storage needs. Thus going from a 512 × 512 matrix to a 1,024 × 1,024 matrix will require a fourfold increase in storage space. In addition, provisions for a larger array processor would have to be made in order to process the data. An array processor is a device that is used in conjunction with the computer to handle large numbers of data in matrix array form such as that found in DSA images. The rate at which images can be acquired, processed through the computer, and recorded on the storage devices must also be considered. On-line storage devices are relatively slow and the ability to acquire images at high rates are compromised in the case of large matrix sizes. Although decreases in matrix size and/or bit depth reduce storage capacity needs, a decrease in image quality also occurs.

Subtraction Modes

Although there is a variety of methods to obtain subtracted images, each method necessitates a "before" and "after" image to accomplish the subtraction process. After successful subtraction, the final image will show only those features unique to the after image.

Mask or Temporal Mode Subtraction

The mask or temporal subtraction mode corresponds to the process previously discussed (Fig. 12A). A sequence of images is obtained before and after the injection of contrast media. One of the before images is selected as a mask image which is then subtracted from the subsequent contrast filled or live images. This permits the visualization of the contrast media as it progresses through the blood vessels with no interference by surrounding soft tissues because are eliminated in the subtraction process. If the patient moved between the onset of the image sequence and the administration of the contrast media, another mask image may be chosen. Because of its speed, the digital approach

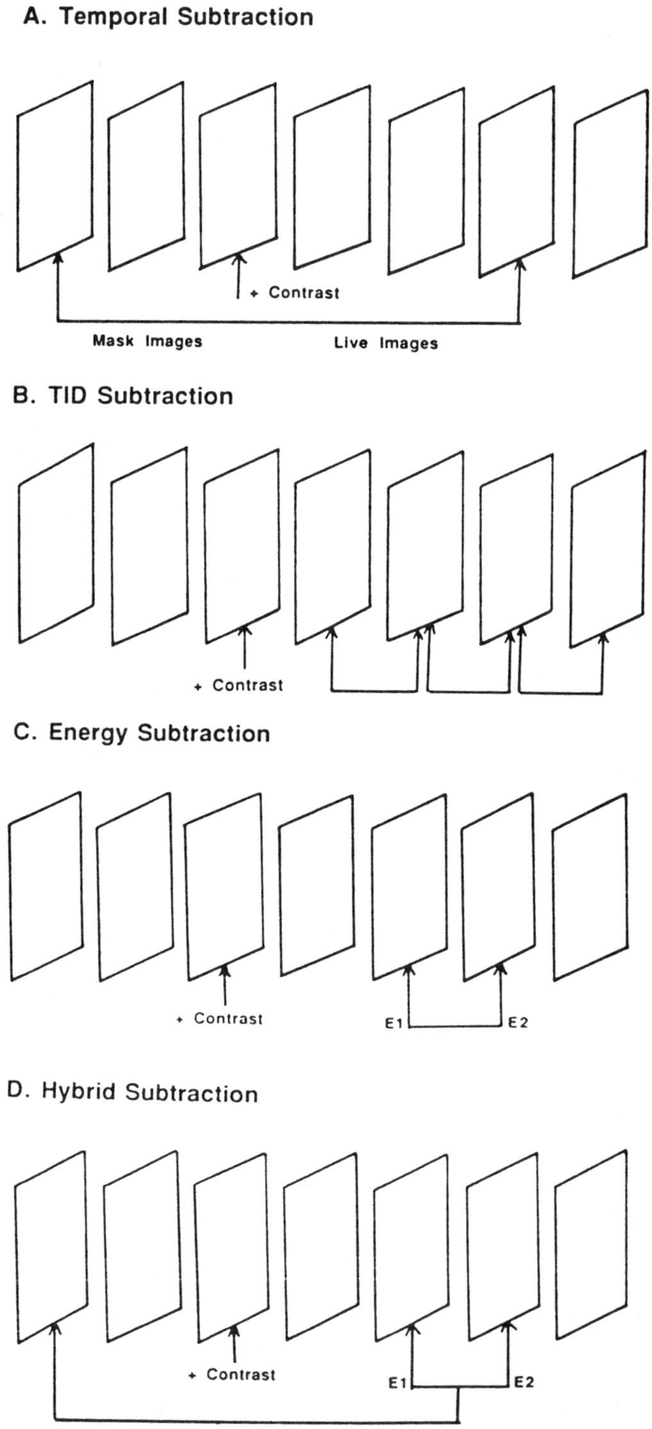
A. Temporal Subtraction
+ Contrast
Mask Images
Live Images
B. TID Subtraction
+ Contrast
C. Energy Subtraction
+ Contrast
E1
E2
D. Hybrid Subtraction
+ Contrast
E1
E2

Figure 12A–D.

decreases the time interval between the mask and live images and provides for a large range of mask/live image combinations yielding digital subtracted images in an almost instantaneous fashion. The major limitation of the mask mode subtraction method is patient motion. Motion limits the ability to register the mask and live images. Achieving an accurate and complete subtraction, therefore, is also limited. An important feature of the digital approach, however, is that image pixels can be shifted in an attempt to undo the effects of motion (Fig 5). Unfortunately, most digital systems are limited to linear shifting up and down and left to right. Patient motion, however, is not linear or in any one single direction. Pixel shifting thus may not always be successful in undoing the effects of motion and is also time consuming.

Time Interval Difference Subtraction (TID)

In TID subtraction one image is subtracted from the very next image in the sequence. This procedure allows for the visualization of the contrast media arriving at a site irrespective of the concentration of the contrast media that had been present immediately prior in time. Although not extensively used clinically, the problem of patient motion is significantly minimized by this approach because the time interval between successive mask and live images is very short. A major disadvantage to this subtraction method is the fact that the full iodine signal is not obtained from each image and therefore the resulting images are of poor quality.

Energy Subtraction

The energy subtraction mode is of significant value in minimizing the problems related to misregistration and motion (Fig. 12C). In this approach the before and after images are obtained within an extremely short time interval of each other and at different energies. The two distinct energy subtraction approaches are: (1) K-edge subtraction and (2) Photoelectric/Compton decomposition.

←

FIGURE 12. **A**: *Temporal Subtraction. Sequence of images is obtained both before (mask image) and after the administration of contrast material (live image). Appropriate subtraction can then be performed.* **B**: *Time Interval Difference (TID). Subtractions are performed between a given image and the image obtained immediately prior in time. This serves to reduce the patient motion problem to a minimum since very little time transpires between images. This approach also subtracts out some of the iodine signal and signal-to-noise ratio worsens.* **C**: *Energy Subtraction. Subtraction is performed between images obtained at relatively high and low energies (E_1 and E_2). This serves to enhance the iodine signal, subtract background structures, and eliminate the motion problem.* **D**: *Hybrid Subtraction. Subtraction is between the energy subtraction image and a precontrast mask. This serves to further minimize whatever soft tissue or bone structures that remain on the energy subtraction image. It does, however, reintroduce a potential motion misregistration problem.*

K-edge Subtraction

Iodine absorbs an extraordinarily large number of x-ray photons with energies just above the binding energy of the electrons in the iodine K shell (K edge). On the other hand, iodine absorbs comparatively few x-ray photons with energies just below the binding energy of the electrons in the iodine K shell. Over this same energy interval anatomic tissues show little if any absorption differences. These facts form the basis for K-edge subtraction. If two images are obtained, one above and one below the K edge of iodine, the image below the K edge will show all the various anatomic structures, but less of the contrast-filled blood vessels. This image below the K edge can serve as a mask image. The image obtained at an energy just above the K edge of iodine will show the contrast-filled blood vessels as well as the various anatomic structures. Therefore, if the two images are subtracted one from the other, the final subtracted image will show only the contrast-filled blood vessels as the soft tissues and bone will be subtracted away or eliminated. One problem associated with the K-edge approach is providing sufficiently intense monochromatic x-ray sources just below and just above the iodine K edge. The energies in an x-ray beam typically are broadly distributed and the various beam filtration strategies often result in unacceptably low x-ray photon levels.[3] There has been some experimental work in using synchrotron particle accelerators to provide monochromatic x-ray beams.[4] Such approaches, however, are not clinically practical at the present time.

Photoelectric/Compton Decomposition

The x-ray absorption of iodine changes significantly between certain ranges such as 85 kVp and 135 kVp. The relatively large difference in absorption for iodine and bone over this energy range is predominantly due to photoelectric interactions (Fig. 13). There is, however, relatively little difference in absorption for the lower atomic number soft tissues which interact predominantly via Compton interactions. As a result, optimal "before" and "after" images are obtained and the iodine signal is greatly enhanced with subtraction (Fig. 12C).

In the dual-energy subtraction methods, patient motion is essentially eliminated as the images to be subtracted are obtained over very short time (milliseconds) intervals. To accomplish energy subtraction, the x-ray equipment must be capable of rapid switching between the two desired kVp. This is a significant requirement, because not all generators are capable of rapidly switching between the two desired kVp. Some energy subtraction approaches also provide for the rapid placement of different filters as the kVp are switched. Filters are used to help shape the x-ray energy distribution so there is a more distinct separation of the x-ray energies above and below the iodine K edge or between low and high kVp. Filters, however, markedly reduce the x-ray intensities, thus image noise and low signal-to-noise ratios become a problem. The separation of energies in the Photoelectric/Compton decomposition approach is never totally com-

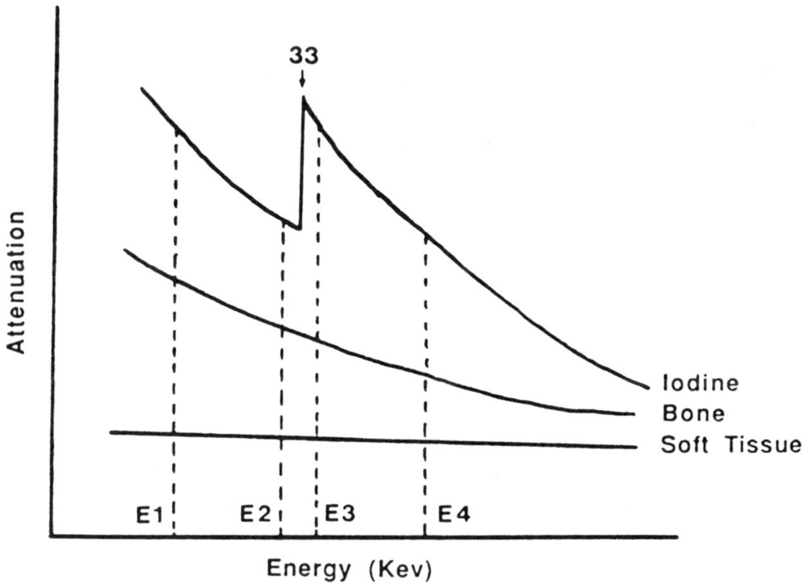

FIGURE 13. Energy subtraction. Generalized x-ray attenuation in iodine and soft tissues. Attenuation in iodine changes significantly over the typical diagnostic x-ray energies. The change in soft tissue attenuation, however, is relatively small while the bone tissue difference, although not as great as for iodine, is greater than that of soft tissue. For iodine a significant difference exists both over a wide range of energies as between E1 and E4, usually corresponding to 85 and 135 kV(p), respectively, and over the short energy interval from just below to just above the K edge (E2 to E3). The photoelectric/Compton decomposition energy subtraction approach exploits the former and K edge subtraction exploits the latter.

plete and, as a result, there will be a faint outline of the contrast vessels on the lower kVp images. In addition, it is not possible to remove both soft tissue and bone simultaneously in the decomposition approach since bone suffers significant photoelectric absorption changes over the 85–135 kVp range. To minimize these effects, *Hybrid* energy subtraction may be utilized (Fig. 12D). In the Hybrid subtraction approach, the first energy-subtracted image is obtained. Then, an image which shows the vessel or bone structure outlines to be eliminated is chosen from the precontrast image sequence. The before-contrast image is used as a mask just as in the standard mask-mode subtraction procedure.

There are important differences between K-edge and Photoelectric/Compton decomposition approaches to accomplish dual-energy subtraction. The K-edge approach ideally requires near monochromatic x-ray beams with energies just below and above the K edge of iodine. These conditions, although possible, are very hard to implement in practice without resorting to signal-robbing filtration techniques. The decomposition approach, on the other hand, uses x-ray beams of low kVp and high kVp. Scatter is more of a problem in the decomposition approach since the high-energy beam produces much more scatter than the low-energy beam. Another problem with the decomposition approach is the significant attenuation of the low kVp beam when passing through thicker parts of the patient. This results in a relatively low photon flux at the detector and consequently a reduction in the signal-to-noise ratio. The advantages of dual-energy subtraction, however, are clearly significant as the problems of patient motion and misregistration are minimized by the use of this technique. In addition, it is important to note that the decomposition approach can provide for selective subtraction independent of atomic number and even for tissues without a distinct K edge. Although this technique is not routinely used in DSA, it has been successful in the selective removal of structures such as bone from a chest radiograph and bowel gas on excretory urography.[5,6]

Signal Filtration Techniques

The subtraction process has been shown to consistently improve the visualization of blood vessels by removing background tissue signals. The subtraction process may be considered a "filtration" process in that unnecessary and unwanted signals have been filtered out while the desired signals have been selected for visualization. The signal theory provides other mathematical techniques for enhancing the desired signal by manipulating the time sequence of images.[7] Examples of this as applied to DSA are matched filtering and recursive filtering. These approaches have the potential of reducing the radiation dose to the patient and enhancing the signal-to-noise ratio, thus improving DSA performance. The interested reader is referred to the literature for more detailed discussions of these approaches.[8–10]

Imaging Performance in DSA

In DSA, as in all imaging modalities, particular concern must be given to the various parameters that affect imaging performance. The important performance parameters fall into four broad categories: (1) image contrast, (2) spatial resolution, (3) noise, and (4) distortions and artifacts. Any one of these parameters alone does not specify the overall performance of an imaging system. Measures combining one or more of these parameters, such as low-contrast resolution and signal-to-noise ratio measures, are therefore used to determine the performance of an imaging system.

Image Contrast

Subject contrast is defined as that which permits a structure to be distinguished from the surrounding structures. This will be determined by the depth or shadow on the image profile, which in turn is due to the relative attenuation of the x-rays as they pass through the tissues. The greater the image depth or subject contrast, the more readily the structure of interest (image contrast) will

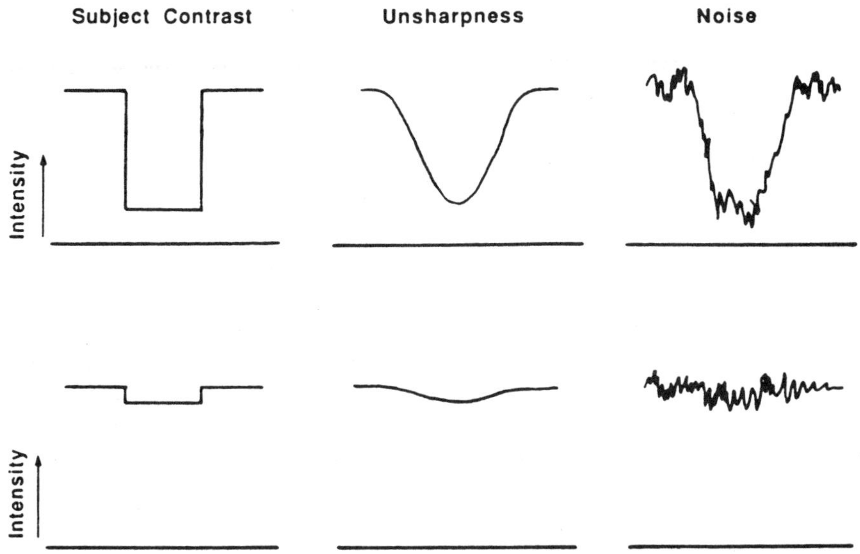

FIGURE 14. **A**: *Series of line profiles having high (top) and low (bottom) subject contrast. Subject contrast of an anatomical structure depends on the capability of that structure to attenuate the beam relative to background tissues.* **B**: *Line profile illustrating the concept of unsharpness that leads to loss of spatial resolution. Note that unsharpness may not drastically affect a high-contrast image but will affect a low-contrast image making it more difficult to distinguish features on the image.* **C**: *Line profile illustrating the effects of image noise. When noise is added, the high-contrast image is still easily distinguished, whereas the presence of noise readily obliterates the low-contrast image.*

be visualized. In general, subject contrast increases when: (1) beam energy decreases (e.g., lower kVp, lower beam filtration), and (2) scatter decreases (e.g., lower beam energy, less patient thickness, smaller field size, larger grid ratios). The final image contrast in DSA will be the result of subtracting whatever subject contrast a blood vessel has from the surrounding background tissue signals. Line profiles with both high and low subject contrast are illustrated in Figure 14A.

Spatial Resolution

Spatial resolution refers to the capability of a system to distinguish fine detail. The image profile illustrated in Figure 14B is noted to have a certain depth as well as unsharpness. The relative spreading around the edges of each image is what is referred to as unsharpness. If the original object were square, then the edges of the image of that object would be expected to be sharp. The presence of image degrading unsharpness is readily manifested by loss of detail along the edges of each object. The sharpness or unsharpness of a vessel will also be influenced by the diameter of the vessel. If an object is very small and has a low subject contrast, then a small amount of unsharpness will easily obliterate the image of the object.

Unsharpness is a particular measure of spatial resolution. The most general and objective measure of spatial resolution, however, is the modulation transfer function (MTF).[11] The MTF describes the resolution response of the system in terms of how the system responds to various sinusoidal frequencies. In practice, however, spatial resolution is characterized by specifying the capability of the system to record a pattern of closely spaced linear objects (bar pattern) in terms of line pairs per millimeter (LPM). The LPM of a system represents the highest frequency of line pairs just discernable.

The effects of the focal spot in DSA are similar to those that occur in general fluoroscopy. Specifically, the smaller the focal spot, the greater the potential image quality. In practice there is a trade-off that must be made, since larger focal spots allow for higher mA and kVp resulting in shorter exposure times with a concomitant decrease in patient motion and an increase in possible frame rates (Fig. 15). It should also be realized that measured focal spot sizes are typically 30% to 50% greater than the manufacturers' stated nominal sizes.

As a rule, image intensifiers have a limiting resolution of 4- to 5-line pairs/mm which is greater than the resolution of the video chain. The video chain is a limiting factor. The spatial resolution can be increased by using the electronic magnification within the image intensifier. The greater the degree of electronic magnification used, the greater the resolution. Specifically, the greater the mag-

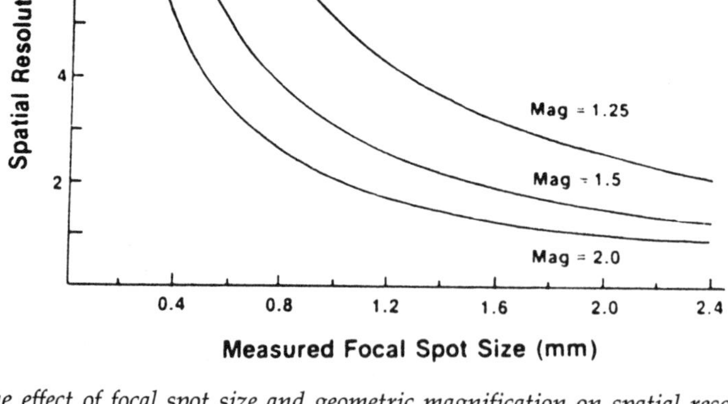

FIGURE 15. The effect of focal spot size and geometric magnification on spatial resolution. Note that progressively higher resolution is possible in line pairs per mm (lp/mm) for smaller focal spot sizes and for smaller magnification. (Adapted with permission from AAPM Report #15, 1985.)

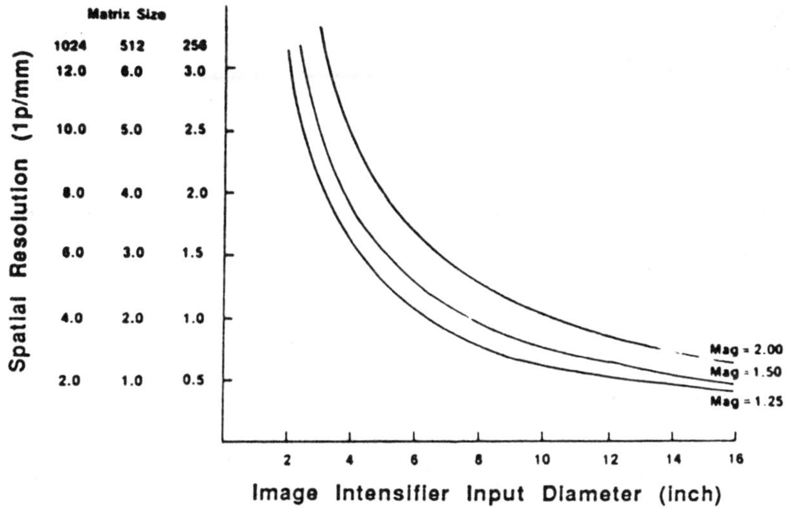

FIGURE 16. *The effect on spatial resolution when combining image intensifier input phosphor diameter, geometric magnification, and matrix size. Note that progressively higher resolution is possible for larger matrix size, smaller image intensifier input diameter, and larger magnification. (Adapted with permission from AAPM Report #15, 1985.)*

nification of small objects, the larger they will appear and thus the better they will be visualized.

Pixel size or display matrix must also be taken into account when determining spatial resolution.[12] Pixel size determines the smallest volume element being imaged in the patient and, as such, forms the theoretical maximum resolution of the system. In electronic magnification techniques, the chosen diameter over which the display matrix is applied will result in significant changes in resolution. For instance, given a fixed matrix size of 512 × 512, the geometrical magnification to 1.25 (which occurs when changing from a 10 in to a 6 in input phosphor) will result in a change in line pairs/mm from approximately 1.2 to 2.2 (Fig. 16). The video chain is usually the limiting factor in the spatial resolution of DSA systems with the governing factors being the electronic focusing and the diameter size of the electronic beam within the video camera. In addition, the optical focusing between the image intensifier output phosphor and the video camera is also important.

Patterns used to determine spatial resolution are referred to as resolution bar patterns (Fig. 17). These patterns consist of alternating strips of lead with equal size spaces. As the strips and spaces progressively become smaller and closer together, their frequency increases. Using such patterns, the typical spatial resolution for an image intensifier video chain is between 1.0- and 2.5-line pairs/mm at the video monitor depending on the size of the input phosphor and display matrix.

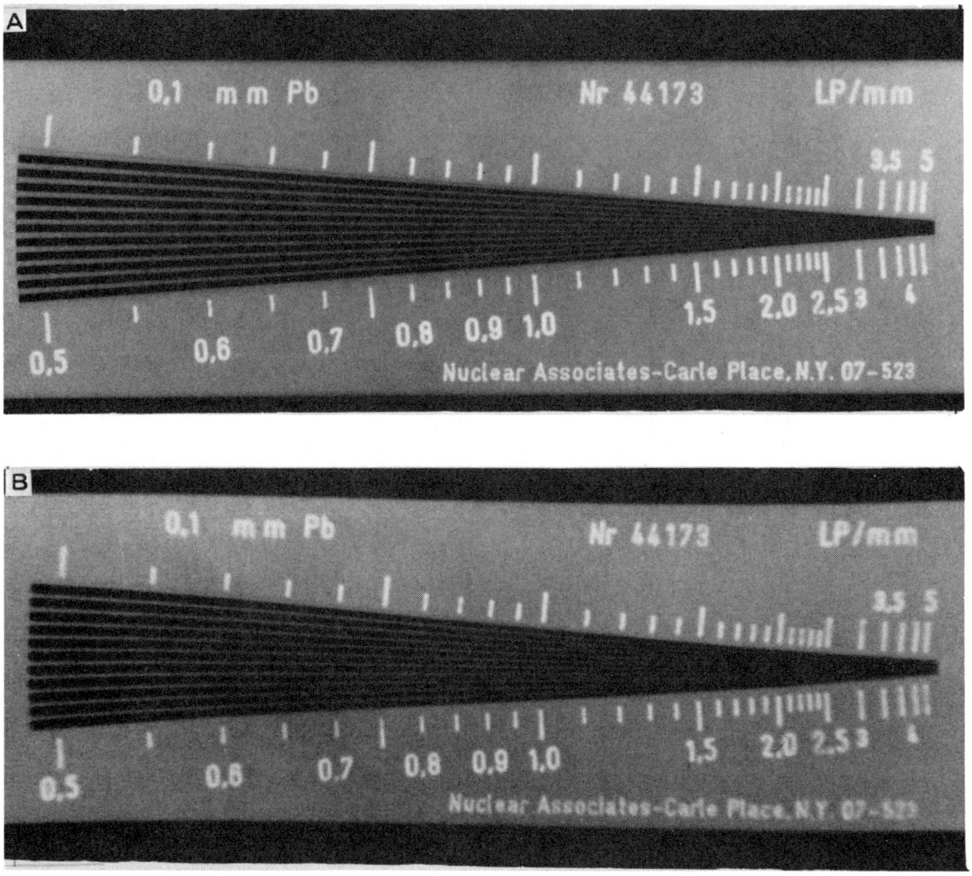

FIGURE 17. Resolution wedge pattern as commonly used to determine spatial resolution of DSA systems. **A**: *Image obtained using radiographic spot film device.* **B**: *Image obtained on 105-mm image-intensified spot camera. Note that greater resolution is available from radiographic spot films compared to image intensified spot films*

Image Noise

The x-ray intensity image profile emerging from the patient is not uniformly flat, but rather has a statistical fluctuation associated with the number of photons at every point of the image. This statistical fluctuation or noise degrades the image. Low-contrast structurs (those that cast a very shallow shadow) are easily lost in the noise (Fig. 14C). High-contrast structures, however, are more visible in the presence of noise. The statistical fluctuation is related to the number of x-ray photons emerging from the patient and is referred to as quantum mottle (QM) or x-ray noise. This particular source of noise is a purely random statistical phenomenon and is entirely dependent on the number of x-ray photons utilized at the image plane. It is expressed by the following equation:

$$\text{Quantum Mottle} = K/\sqrt{N}$$

N is equal to the number of x-ray photons utilized in the image and K is a proportionality constant. The equation above states that: (1) if the number of x-ray photons utilized in the image is doubled, the quantum mottle will be reduced by a factor of $1/\sqrt{2}$ or by 0.71; (2) to reduce quantum mottle by a factor of 2, the radiation dose to the patient would have to be quadrupled; and (3) if the number of photons arriving at the image plane is reduced by a factor of 2, the quantum mottle will be increased by a factor of 1.41.

In addition to quantum mottle there are a number of other sources of image degrading noise in DSA including electronic noise introduced by the image intensifier and video chain as well as by the storage devices, video camera noise, and video time jitter (pixel not placed at a consistent point in the image). Random process noise such as quantum mottle and electronic noise in the image chain cause fluctuations from frame to frame and from pixel to pixel and represent the principle image degrading factor. In practice, the ideal should be governed by quantum mottle only and not by electronic noise.

Noise is also introduced at the ADC when the image is divided into finite size pixels. This results in a loss of information and in the formation of images composed of a series of distracting visible square pixels. The resulting checkerboard pattern becomes more apparent as the size of these square pixels increases.

Fixed-pattern noise refers to nonrandomly produced noise. Sources of fixed-pattern noise include manufacturing variations in a number of the components of the system such as: the uniformity and granularity of the image intensifier input and output phosphors; TV camera target imperfections; and ADC step size uniformity. Interestingly, if there is a sufficient amount of a fixed-pattern noise it is usually not a limiting factor as the noise will be present in the before and the after images and will be removed in the subtraction process.

Frame Averaging

Frame averaging is a method by which noise is minimized. In this method, successive image frames are added, resulting in an increase in the number of x-ray photons making up each image and thus a reduction in quantum mottle. Quantum mottle is reduced because random noise fluctuations tend to be equally distributed about some average value and will be canceled out as successive images are added frame by frame. At the same time, the desired real image signal will be consistently added and reinforced. The final result is that the signal-to-noise ratio is considerably enhanced.

Frame averaging also can be used to reduce the radiation dose to the patient. Although quantum mottle increases with lower radiation doses, the effect of quantum mottle can be minimized if frame averaging is utilized. A disadvantage to frame averaging is the increased potential for motion misregistration artifacts, since the use of more frames increases the time interval over which images are integrated.

Signal-to-Noise Ratio

It is very useful to combine into a ratio the contrast signal strength available and the noise present in the system. This ratio, the signal-to-noise ratio (SNR) is a fundamental performance parameter of the system. The SNR is defined as follows:

$$\text{SNR} = \frac{\text{Contrast Signal}}{\text{Noise}}$$

The contrast signal noted in the above equation is the signal from a contrast-filled blood vessel from which the neighboring background signal is subtracted. The contrast signal, therefore, represents the subtracted image signal. The value for the subtracted image signal is found by placing a region of interest (ROI) over the vessel being studied and subtracting the displayed value for this region from the value displayed when a region of interest is placed over an adjacent background area. The noise number is the pixel standard deviation over the background image within the ROI. All commercially available DSA units incorporate capabilities for defining regions of interest of different sizes and for performing averaging and standard deviation calculations.

The importance of SNR is recognized when the image signal is electronically amplified in order to improve detection of image features. If the image signal was originally of high SNR, then very small features can be obtained from the image. If the image signal was of low SNR, then amplification results in the noise being amplified while the features of interest are easily lost.

Low-Contrast Resolution

Resolution, subject contrast, and noise all affect image visualization in DSA. The performance parameter that accounts for these factors is the low-contrast resolution of the system. Contrast resolution measures the capabilities of the system to detect and record the presence of low levels of iodine for a given vessel diameter. The best system is one that, for a given iodine concentration in a blood vessel (subject contrast), demonstrates a vessel of very small diameter at the lowest possible radiation dose to the patient. It is common to specify a contrast resolution of 1 mm at 1% subject contrast for a 1 mR exposure to the face of the image intensifier. It is necessary to specify the milliroentgen exposure, because the exposure determines the x-ray photon level which, in turn, controls the noise level of the system. As noted previously, noise critically affects the size and contrast of the structures that can be visualized. It is important to note that a given system may be capable of demonstrating a blood vessel with a diameter of 1 mm at 1% contrast but only at a high-radiation exposure to the patient. Low-contrast resolution must be stated with the radiation exposure clearly specified. The exposure of 1 mR is specified at the face of the image intensifier and does not specify the actual dose received by the patient; the skin dose, in fact, may be 100 times more.

The low-contrast resolution of the DSA process is significantly greater than that in conventional film angiography. This is of great significance as it allows angiography to be performed by means of intravenous injections of contrast media or the use of reduced and safer doses of contrast media for intra-arterial injections.

Low-contrast resolution depends on the contrast signal arriving at the image intensifier and the capability of the video chain to detect and display this signal. The contrast signal, in turn, depends on the iodine concentration in the patient, the vessel size, and the original subject contrast. Many factors affect subject contrast such as beam quality (kVp and filtration combination), the presence of scatter as determined by patient thickness, field size, and grid ratio. The veiling glare of the video monitor results in the loss of contrast signal. The glare is due to the background glare on the monitor face and is responsible for undercutting and obscuring the signal areas on the monitor.

The degree of geometric and electronic magnification employed also is of importance. With magnification, objects appear larger and thus less subject to the spatial resolution limits of the system. Magnification also provides for smaller volume pixels. Lastly, quantum mottle and system noise (the signal-to-noise ratio) are crucial in determining the final low-contrast resolution performance of the system. In general, the lower the quantum mottle, the greater the low contrast performance of the system. Increasing the radiation exposure and/or increasing pixel sizes will reduce quantum mottle levels.

Distortions and Artifacts

DSA performance is also affected by the presence of distortions and artifacts. A distortion such as spatial nonuniformity can enter via various optical effects such as the pin cushion distortion. This is due to the curved input phosphor surface and vignetting effects.[13] Nonlinearities in the image intensifier electron optics and optical lenses may also introduce spatial distortions.

Contrast nonlinearity distortions may also result from improper logarithmic processing of widely varying signals such as those from osseous and nonosseous structures. Logarithmic processing is very important in DSA, since it allows the contrast signal to be directly proportional to the iodine content and independent of the transmitted x-ray beam. Utilizing logarithmic processing, quantitative physiologic measurements related to the cardiovascular system can be performed and the appearance of the blood vessels will be independent of the thickness of the patient.

References

1. Kruger RA, Riederer SJ: *Basic Concepts of Subtraction Angiography*, Boston, G.K. Hall Medical Publ., 1984.
2. Brody WR: *Digital Radiography*, New York, Raven Press, 1984.

3. Misttreta CA, Ort ME, Kelcz E, Cameron JR, Siedband MP, Crummy AB: Absorption edge fluoroscopy using quasi-monoenergetic x-ray beams. *Invest Radiol* 8:402–412, 1973.
4. Rubenstein E, Hughes EB, Campbell LE, Hofstadter R, Kirk RL, Krolicki TS: Synchotron radiation and its application to digital subtraction angiography. *Proc SPIE* 314:42–49, 1981.
5. Brody WR, Cassel DM, Sommer FG, Lehmann LA, Macovski A, Alvarez RE, Pelc NJ, Riederer SJ, Hall AL: Dual energy projection radiography: Initial clinical experience. *Am J Roentgenol* 137:201–205, 1981.
6. Sommer FG, Brody WR, Gross D, Macovski A, Hall A, Pelc NJ: Excretory urography using dual energy scanned radiography. *Radiology* 141:529–532, 1981.
7. Kruger RA, Nelson JA: Digital angiography using bandpass filtration: Searching for gold. *Diagn Imaging* 24–29, 1982.
8. Riederer SJ, Enzmann DR, Hall AL, Pelc NJ, DJang WT: The application of matched filtering to x-ray exposure reduction in digital subtraction angiography: Clinical results. *Radiology* 146:249–254, 1983.
9. Riederer SJ, Enzmann DR, Hall AL, Pelc NJ, DJang WT: Technical characteristics of matched filtering in digital subtraction angiography. *Med Phys* 10:209–217, 1983.
10. Kruger RA, Miller FJ, Nelson JA, Liu PY, Bateman W: Digital subtraction angiography using temporal bandpass filter. *Radiology* 145:315–320, 1982.
11. Villafana T: Advantages, Limitation and Significance of the Modulation Transfer Function in Radiologic Practice. *Curr Probl Diag Radiol* 7, number 10, July/August, 1982.
12. *Performance Evaluation and Quality Assurance in Digital Subtraction Angiography*. Am Assoc of Physicists in Medicine Report 15, 1985.
13. Curry TS, Dowdey JE, Murry RC: *Christensen's Introduction to the Physics of Diagnostic Radiology* 3rd ed. Philadelphia, Lea and Febiger, 1984, 198–199.

Chapter 2

Techniques of Digital Subtraction Angiography

ARINA VAN BREDA

Introduction

Digital subtraction angiography represents a major advance in vascular imaging technology. As such, it should be considered an integral part of contemporary angiography. Its advantages are particularly pertinent when performing pediatric angiographic studies. These advantages include: increased contrast sensitivity and marked improvement in the overall speed of the angiographic studies, which results in a great increase in patient comfort and a decrease in patient morbidity during angiographic studies. However, as with standard angiography, optimum image quality and patient care can be obtained only with exacting attention to detail. Initially, digital subtraction angiography promised to allow angiographic studies without angiographic skills; this has clearly proven not to be the case. Moreover, good digital subtraction studies may be more difficult to obtain than standard studies. The purpose of this chapter is to introduce some basic techniques which will help provide optimum digital subtraction angiographic studies. Much of this assumes "state of the art" digital subtraction equipment integrated completely into a fully equipped angiographic laboratory. Current digital equipment should include on-line image processing, rapid image acquisition and retrieval, "user friendly" postprocessing procedures, a high signal-to-noise ratio, and rapid frame-rate acquisition (12–30 frames/sec). An image intensifier (12–14 inches) with a large field of view is preferable, though less mandatory in pediatric patients than in adults. The imaging system should be a C- or L/U-arm configuration to allow complex angulation without moving the patient.[1]

Digital Subtraction Imaging in Infants and Children, edited by Eric N. Faerber. Mount Kisco, New York: Futura Publishing Company, Inc., © 1989.

Patient and Case Selection

Digital subtraction angiography may prove to be the sole imaging modality required to provide complete anatomic information; in other instances, digital subtraction angiography (DSA) may be used to supplement a standard angiographic study. Selection of imaging modalities must be made on clinical grounds; however, digital subtraction angiography should be employed whenever feasible because of its obvious advantages. These include greater contrast sensitivity, decreased contrast requirement, increased speed of studies, and decreased cost due to decreased film usage. Since neither imaging modality may be diagnostic by itself, the angiographer should be prepared to perform either study in order to obtain complete diagnostic information. It is generally preferable to obtain all of the necessary anatomic information during a single study if this can be performed without undue risk to the patient.

Case selection in digital subtraction angiography should be based on a thorough understanding of both the advantages and limitations of digital subtraction technology. In the pediatric patient population, the following factors are especially important: minimizing contrast volume, minimizing patient discomfort, decreasing the overall time of the examination, and as with all imaging studies, optimizing image quality. All of these issues but the latter are obtainable with digital. Excellent anatomic information can be obtained with a fraction of the contrast volumes required with standard angiography. This is especially important with smaller patients. It must be remembered, however, that the resolution of digital systems will not compare to standard angiography being approximately 1.5 line pairs/mm versus 4 line pairs/mm with standard angiography. In addition, it must be remembered that digital studies are markedly degraded by motion and therefore the body part being studied should be immobilized if possible. This generally presents no problem in the extremities. In the chest, however, respiratory motion and cardiac motion can seriously degrade image quality; in the abdomen respiratory motion and bowel peristalsis may provide sources of serious image degradation. Some of the motion artifact may be avoided by judicious use of sedation and/or general anesthesia. It is preferable to employ only sedation if at all possible. Bowel peristalsis may be partly addressed by the use of intravenous glucagon, or by gentle compression devices.[2]

The imaging modality best suited to a given study will depend in part on the type of anatomic information desired. Major vascular structures can be very satisfactorily imaged by digital subtraction techniques, whereas standard angiography or magnification angiography will be required for smaller vessel detail. For example, digital subtraction angiography can demonstrate major abnormalities in the thoracic and abdominal aorta and their major branches. Major vascular occlusions, aneurysms, and arterial venous malformations will be readily identified. Small vessel abnormalities, i.e., intrarenal vascular detail, intracranial vascular changes, or detection of tumor vessels, will require the higher resolution offered by standard angiography.

Techniques

Digital subtraction angiography may be performed from intravenous or intra-arterial approach; the latter may be nonselective or selective in nature.[3] The technique should be chosen to provide maximal anatomic information at minimal risk to the patient. Major vascular abnormalities can be readily identified by intravenous digital subtraction angiography which has a lower morbidity because of the avoidance of arterial puncture; however, it does require larger contrast volumes than intra-arterial studies. The higher contrast sensitivity afforded by digital subtraction techniques will allow satisfactory vascular opacification with an intravenous injection with contrast volume similar to those used for standard arteriography during an arterial injection. The relative contrast sensitivity is further increased by the smaller size of the pediatric patient, allowing much better image quality for correspondingly lower doses of contrast.

Intravenous Digital Subtraction Angiography

The venous approach to digital subtraction is preferred in children as it avoids the need for arterial puncture which has a higher rate of complication in children.[4] Intravenous studies can be performed from several approaches; a peripheral intravenous line of satisfactory caliber may allow a bolus injection sufficient to satisfactorily perform digital subtraction studies in a nonperipherally vasoconstricted patient. Peripheral injections should be performed through short intravenous catheters rather than needles that may lead to extravasation and do not allow a sufficiently rapid injection.[2] Peripheral injection may avoid the necessity of central venous line placement. If this must be performed, it can be from either a jugular or femoral venous route percutaneously or venous cut down. In neonates, central venous transumbilical lines can be used as long as documentation of a satisfactory catheter position is obtained prior to contrast injections. For intravenous injections, nondilute contrast material is used. The overall rates and total volumes of the injections will vary depending on the patient's size, cardiac output, and the anatomic structure being studied. As a rough guide, ⅓–½ cc/lb/injection can be used.[2,3] The key factor in obtaining good image quality is ensuring a bolus contrast delivery such that maximum opacification of the vascular system can be obtained at a given point in time. A better bolus can be obtained with central venous injections as opposed to peripheral venous injections.

Imaging Techniques During Digital Subtraction

Positioning

Every attempt should be made to obtain satisfactory positioning of the patient with adequate immobilization of the body part being studied, otherwise motion artifact will make images uninterpretable. Generally, all that is required are gentle restraint devices accompanied by sedative drugs. It is highly preferable to allow the patient to remain stationary and as undisturbed as possible during the examination and therefore a C-arm or L/U-arm configuration of the imaging equipment is preferential to the stationary overhead tube. As some digital subtraction studies in children will be performed by the intravenous route and because the interpretation of these studies may be made difficult by overlap of many vascular structures, the ability to do multiple oblique views to best "lay out" the anatomy is strongly preferred. Because there is no reduction in radiation exposure during digital subtraction angiography compared with standard angiography, it is essential to ensure adequate patient shielding during the procedures. The total radiation dose, however, will be less than that received from standard angiography because of decreased fluoroscopy time.

Contrast Media

For venous digital studies, undiluted contrast (370 mg iodine/mL) should be used in doses as outlined above. Every effort should be made to keep contrast totals to a minimum, especially in the very young patient. After an initial injection, contrast doses may need to be adjusted up or down. In seriously ill children, especially those with hemodynamic compromise, nonionic or low osmolality agents should be used because of the lower incidence of hemodynamic effects with these agents.[6] All premature infants should be given these low-osmolality agents to avoid the hyperosmolality that can occur with standard contrast agents. In larger children, the need for low-osmolality contrast should be determined on a case by case basis. Patients with the following problems should always be given low-osmolality agents: congestive failure, sickle cell anemia or other hemoglobinopathies, elevated pulmonary artery pressure, or history of prior severe contrast reaction to standard agents.[7,8] Low-osmolality contrast also has the significant advantage of producing less patient discomfort during injections. In older children who are being studied with sedation only, this may allow improved image quality during venous digital studies because of the lower likelihood of motion and subsequent image degradation. Low-osmolality contrast only should be used in standard extremity arteriography in awake or sedated patients because of the severe pain associated with standard contrast.

During intra-arterial injections, dilute contrast is used. Dilution of standard osmolality contrast will reduce its osmolality to acceptable levels and obviates the advantage of low osmolality contrast use. In small children ⅓ or ¼ part contrast diluted with saline should provide satisfactory image quality; this will depend to some degree on the contrast sensitivity of the digital system being used. With arterial digital studies it is again important to deliver the contrast in a bolus with sufficient volumes injected to completely opacify the vascular system being studied. As a general rule, ½–⅔ the total volume of contrast used in standard angiographic studies is sufficient (i.e. if 12 cc is normally used for an injection, we would use 6 cc of dilute contrast for the corresponding digital study). Again, this will have to be varied based on the blood flow in the organ being studied, the patient's cardiac output, and the degree of vascular detail necessary.

In all patients, total contrast volumes during the study should be limited to 4 cc/kg.

Patient Monitoring

Overall patient care during any angiographic study is the responsibility of the radiologist and in conjunction with the anesthesiologist if sedation or general anesthesia is being administered. All patients should be well hydrated prior to studies; an intravenous line should be placed during the study to administer fluids and drugs as necessary. In patients undergoing venous studies, the same catheter can be used for both contrast and fluid administration. All patients should have ECG monitoring. Temperature monitoring should be performed in smaller children with appropriate measures taken to avoid chilling the patient. Nursing care is an important component of the angiographic environment; preferably a nurse with critical care skills and speciality training in radiology and interventional procedures should be available to assist in patient monitoring during the procedure and postprocedure care.

After the procedure, the angiographer should ensure that adequate hemostasis is achieved and that orders are given for hydration of the patient. Outpatients should be observed for 2–4 hours after the procedure and released after reevaluation by the radiologist. Although arterial digital studies are frequently performed on an outpatient basis in adults, only venous studies should be performed on an outpatient basis in children, and then only in older children in whom the likelihood of complication is lower.

Conclusion

Digital subtraction imaging is a valuable technique that can be of great advantage in vascular imaging of patients of all ages. It requires careful attention to technique to provide optimum image quality, but can significantly lower the morbidity of vascular imaging, especially in the pediatric population. The best image quality requires state-of-the art digital equipment, careful patient selection, and a high level of patient care; with these ingredients digital subtraction angiography warrants a prominent place in pediatric imaging techniques.

References

1. Van Breda A, Katzen BT: *Digital Subtraction Angiography*. Thorofare, NY, Slack Inc., 1986.

2. Wagner ML, Singleton EB, Egan ME: Digital subtraction angiography in children. AJR 140:127–133, 1983.
3. Amundson GM, Wesenberg RL, Mueller DL, Reid RH: Pediatric digital subtraction angiography. *Radiology* 153:649–654, 1984.
4. Hurwitz RA, Franken EA, Girod DA, et al: Angiographic determination of arterial patency after percutaneous catheterization in infants and small children. *Circulation* 56:102–105, 1977.
5. Gordon DH, Kasner G, Haller JO, Yoon JJ: Transumbilical selective angiography in the newborn. *Radiology* 125:248–249, 1977.
6. Wolf GL: Safer, more expensive iodinated contrast agents; How do we decide. *Radiology* 159:557–558, 1986.
7. White RI, Halden WJ: Liquid gold: Low osmolality contrast media. *Radiology* 159:559–560, 1986.
8. McClennan BL: Low osmolality contrast media premises and promises. *Radiology* 162:1–8, 1987.

Chapter 3

Intra-Arterial Digital Subtraction Angiography

PHILIP STANLEY

Introduction

Visualization of the arterial circulation in children is possible with arteriography using a percutaneously introduced catheter with the image being recorded either conventionally on film screen combinations or using a digital technique. Although intravenous digital subtraction angiography was heralded as an effective replacement for conventional catheter arteriography, it has not lived up to its early promise and is now reserved for special circumstances.

As discussed in Chapter 2, digital subtraction angiography offers many advantages over conventional film screen combinations. In intra-arterial digital angiography, the image recorded digitally with an intra-arterial catheter is instantly available in the subtracted form and requires smaller volumes of less concentrated contrast medium. In children, it has particular advantages in reducing the overall time of the examination, thus minimizing the potential complications from contrast load and arterial catheterization. The exposure is usually less than with conventional films, depending upon the image intensifier modes selected. Some of the disadvantages encountered in pediatric arterial applications include some loss of resolution, a field of view limited by the size of the image intensifier, and susceptibility of the image to degradation as a result of patient movement. In addition, careful coning and masking are required to minimize flare from areas of low attenuation, e.g., the lungs and bowel gas.

Intra-arterial digital angiography can be used to complement standard film imaging or in many circumstances can replace conventional techniques. The various applications of pediatric, digital, intra-arterial angiography will be described below.

Digital Subtraction Imaging in Infants and Children, edited by Eric N. Faerber. Mount Kisco, New York: Futura Publishing Company, Inc., © 1989.

Aortic Arch Anomalies

In the newborn with an umbilical arterial catheter in the thoracic aorta, an excellent examination of the aortic arch and major branches may be obtained by the hand injection of 3 cc of nonionic contrast. For patients with esophageal atresia where it is essential to demonstrate the side of the aortic arch prior to repair, this can be easily accomplished (Fig. 1). In patients with congenital vascular malformations of the neck (Fig. 2) or with pulmonary sequestration in whom the arterial blood supply must be identified, umbilical catheter injections will give sufficient visualization so that a therapeutic decision can be made with confidence.

For complex anomalies of the aortic arch, such as aortic rings, intravenous digital has been useful in some studies.[1] However, for the detail necessary to identify the individual aortic components and their branches, we prefer selective arterial catheterization using digital technique in entirety (Fig. 3). For this procedure, the correct tube angulation and an apparatus capable of complex angular motion are essential. A digital camera mounted on a C- or L/U-arm is the easiest method of obtaining these projections without moving the patient (Fig. 4).

Head and Neck Arteriography

Arteriography is still performed in children for the investigation of trauma, vascular disease, aneurysms, arteriovenous malformations, and some tumors. Digital subtraction angiography has the advantage that diagnostic imaging of the intracranial circulation may be obtained via aortic injections. This diminishes the risk of selective catheterization in patients who already have compromised circulation (Fig. 5). Some loss of detail by the digital technique has not altered the diagnostic quality of the exam. However, for fine detail without superimposition of other vessels, selective catheterization is required (Fig. 6). Comparative studies in adults have shown that the digital is more effective in showing tumor blush and the venous phase than conventional studies provided there is no patient movement.[2] Digital imaging has the advantage that multiple projections can be rapidly performed and viewed. For arteriovenous malformations and aneurysms, digital gives sufficient detail prior to therapeutic intervention (Fig. 7). In addition, a mobile C-arm carrying digital can be moved into the surgical suite to assist the surgeon in surgical obliteration of an aneurysm or an arteriovenous malformation not suitable for radiologic intervention. For tumors, digital will demonstrate the arterial blood supply prior to surgery or therapeutic embolization or infusion (Fig. 8).

Spine and Bronchial Arteriography

Spinal arteriography is performed prior to therapy in children with suspected arteriovenous malformations of the spine and children with large tumors involving the aorta. In the latter group, it is essential to demonstrate the level of the artery of the Adamkiewicz before mobilizing the aorta or performing therapeutic embolization (Fig. 9). Bronchial arteriography is performed most frequently in patients with cystic fibrosis who are having massive hemoptysis prior to therapeutic occlusion. Intra-arterial digital is useful in identifying the bronchial artery and monitoring the embolization. Also, hypertrophic bronchial arteries seen with cyanotic heart disease may be obliterated using transcatheter embolization after surgical correction of the basic cardiac anomaly.

Abdominal Angiography

Provided the field of view is sufficient, the abdominal aorta and major vessels can be easily imaged with intra-arterial digital technique. The initial exam can be performed with just a dilator (Fig. 10). Digital is most useful if selective injections are performed. If there is minimal motion, the venous phase can also be examined. For patients who require extensive tumor resection, digital will enable the exam to be performed rapidly and effectively (Fig. 11). For the demonstration of the source of GI bleeding and successful embolization, digital is very effective. In patients with renal artery disease in either the native or transplant kidney, digital is often sufficient in itself to demonstrate the vascular abnormality (Fig. 12) or to show the correct degree of obliquity for the final conventional film screen examination.[3] Intra-arterial digital has a role in the demonstration of portal hypertension (Fig. 13).[4] However, with respiratory movement and peristalsis, there can be deterioration in the late venous images of the superior mesenteric artery injection. Usually the splenic vein will be visualized with the celiac axis injection. In addition, splenoportography can be imaged using digital subtraction techniques thus eliminating the need for conventional film screen recording of the image.

The vascular complications of liver transplantation include occlusion, stenosis, and aneurysm formation.[5] The patency of the anastomosis may be assessed by intravenous digital, but for fine detail intra-arterial injection is required. For this purpose digital will often suffice.

Peripheral Angiography

For the demonstration of trauma, tumors, and angiomatous malformation, digital subtraction has many advantages provided the limb is adequately masked to avoid flare from the air adjacent to the soft tissues. As an adjunct to embolization for AVM, intra-arterial digital subtraction is irreplaceable.

Pulmonary Arteriography

Provided there is selective placement of the catheter, excellent visualization of the pulmonary artery will be achieved. There is, however, considerable loss of detail if the catheter is placed in the right atrium or right ventricle. Pulmonary emboli, the effect of radiation and chemotherapy, and arteriovenous shunts will be demonstrated.

Interventional

Intra-arterial interventional radiology (angioplasty, therapeutic infusion, and embolization (Fig. 14)) requires frequent imaging and potentially excessive contrast loads. With digital, the time of the procedure and contrast load is re-

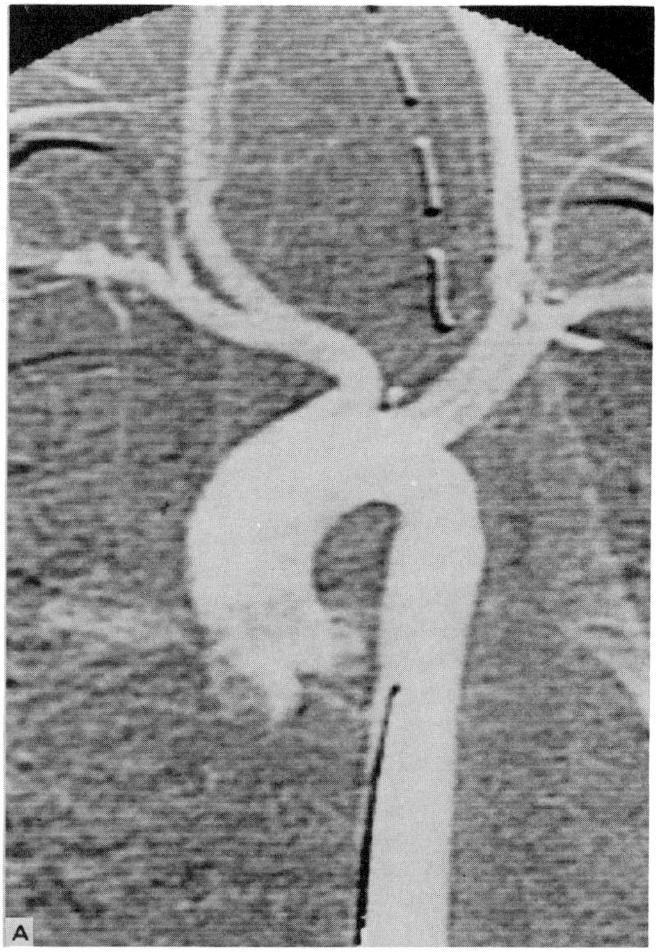

FIGURE 1. *Aortogram of a newborn with esophageal atresia. Injection of 3 cc of dilute nonionic contrast medium with digital recording of the image demonstrates excellent visualization of the aorta. The carotid arteries are displaced laterally by a distended esophagus with a drainage tube in situ. The aortic arch and major branches are normal.*

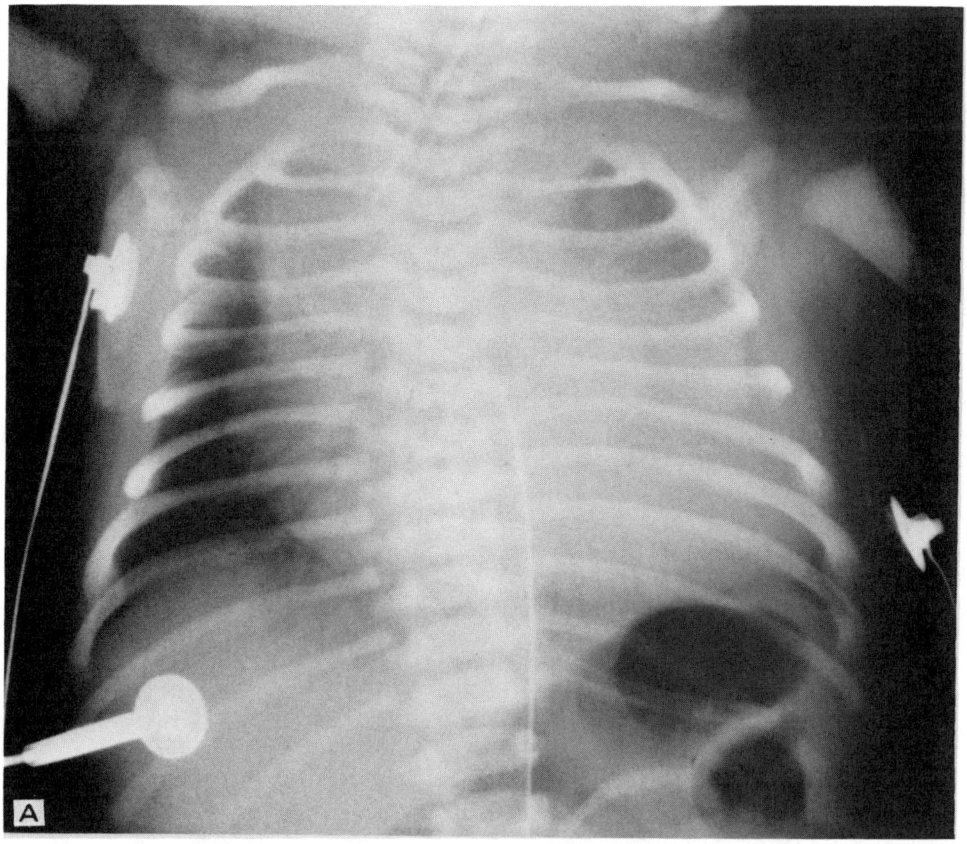

FIGURE 2. **A**: *Chest x-ray of a newborn with a large soft tissue mass occupying the right side of the neck. There is cardiomegaly. The tip of the umbilical arterial catheter is at T6;* **B**: *Contrast injection through the umbilical arterial catheter demonstrates hypertrophy of the innominate and right common carotid arteries;* **C**: *Later phase of the examination demonstrates a vascular mass occupying the right side of the neck with a dilated draining vein.*

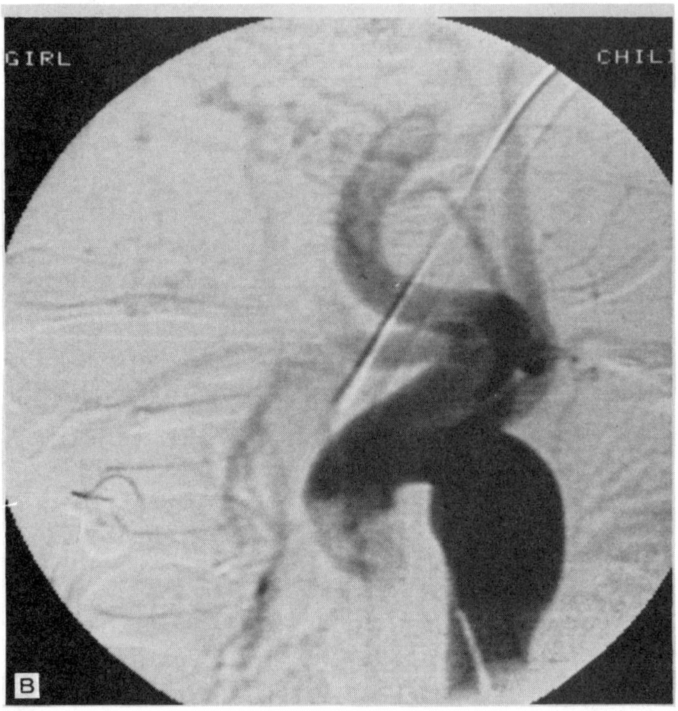

Figure 2B.

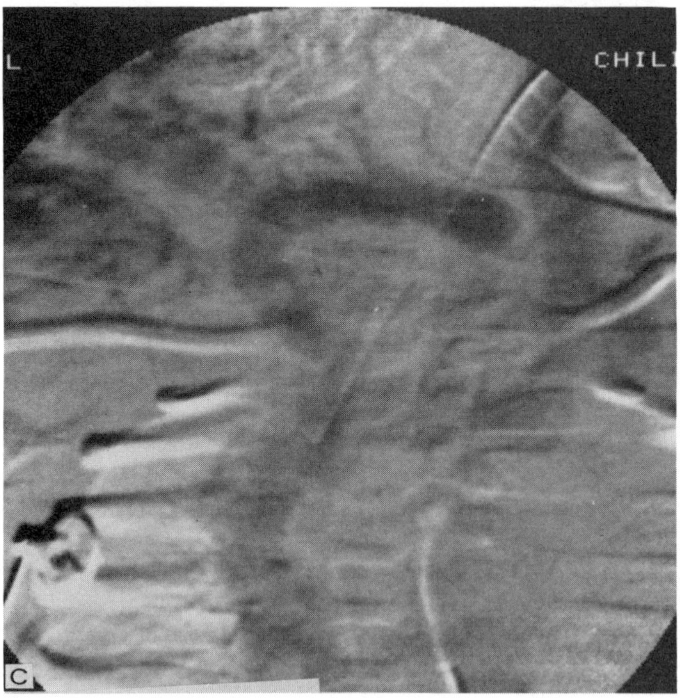

Figure 2C.

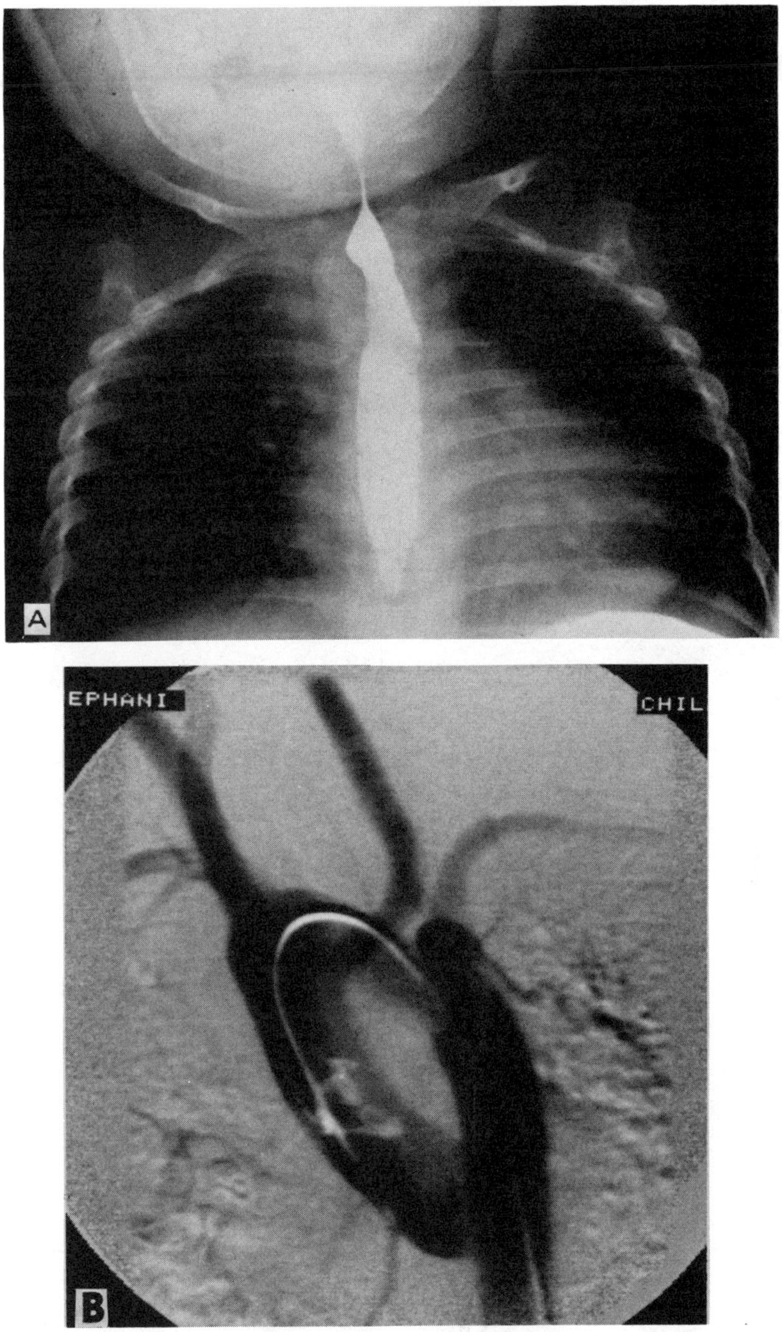

FIGURE 3. **A**: *Esophagram of a two year old with wheezing. There is a right sided aortic arch with posterior impression on the aorta which was better seen on the lateral view;* **B**: *Digital aortogram demonstrates a right-sided ascending aorta with a retroesophageal arch and a left-sided descending aorta. The first branch is the left carotid. There is a diverticulum at the origin of the left subclavian. A ligamentum between the left pulmonary artery and the diverticulum completed the ring. This was easily divided at surgery.*

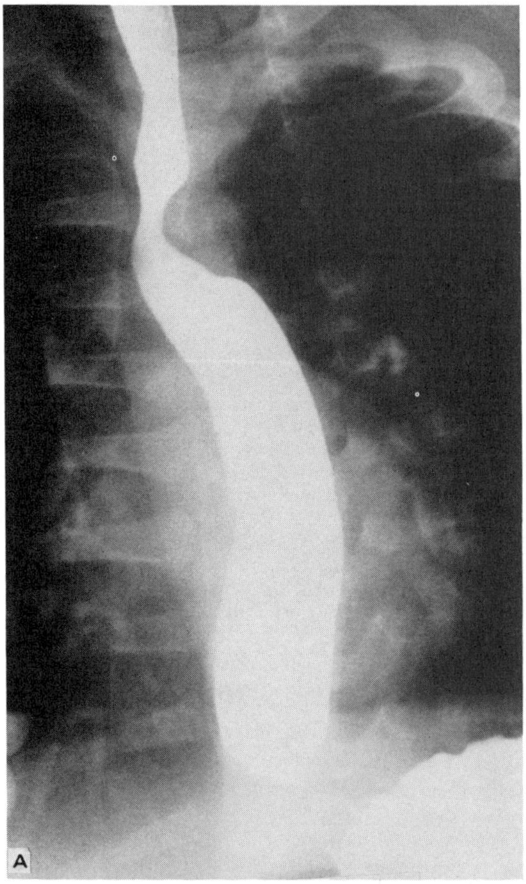

Figure 4A. *Barium swallow of a four month old with wheezing and recurrent pneumonia. There is compression of the upper esophagus by a presumed double aortic arch.*

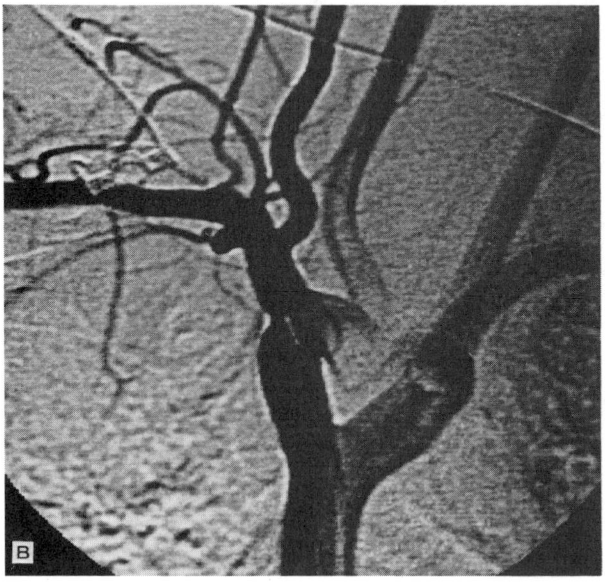

Figure 4B. *Digital aortogram with selective catheterization of the dorsal right component. This exam demonstrates the two dorsal components of the double aortic arch. The left dorsal component was divided with complete relief of the patient's symptoms.*

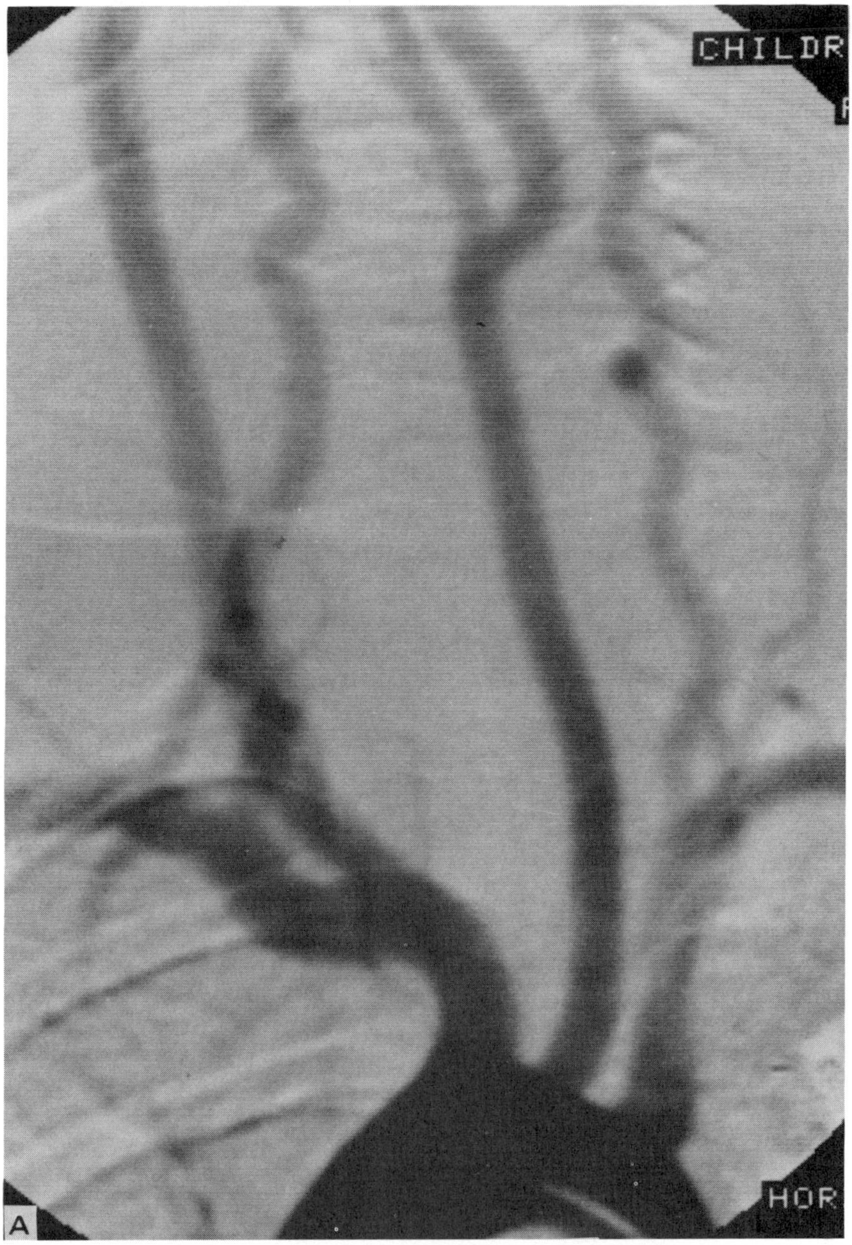

FIGURE 5. **A**: *Aortogram of a patient with sickle cell disease with a stroke. No abnormality has been demonstrated in the origin of the aortic vessels;* **B**: *Head study with an aortic injection demonstrates bilateral occlusion of the anterior cerebral arteries and narrowing of the right internal carotid in the intercavernous course;* **C**: *Later phase demonstrates collateral vessels supplying the territory of the anterior cerebral.*

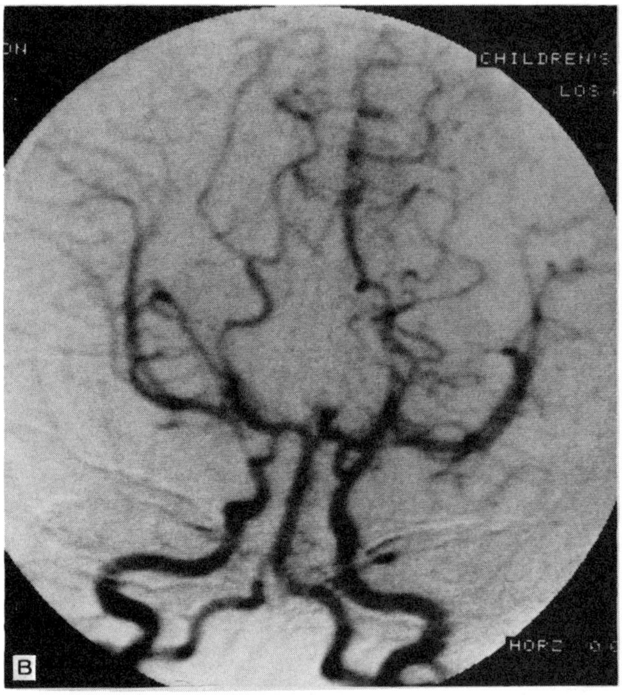

FIGURE 5B.

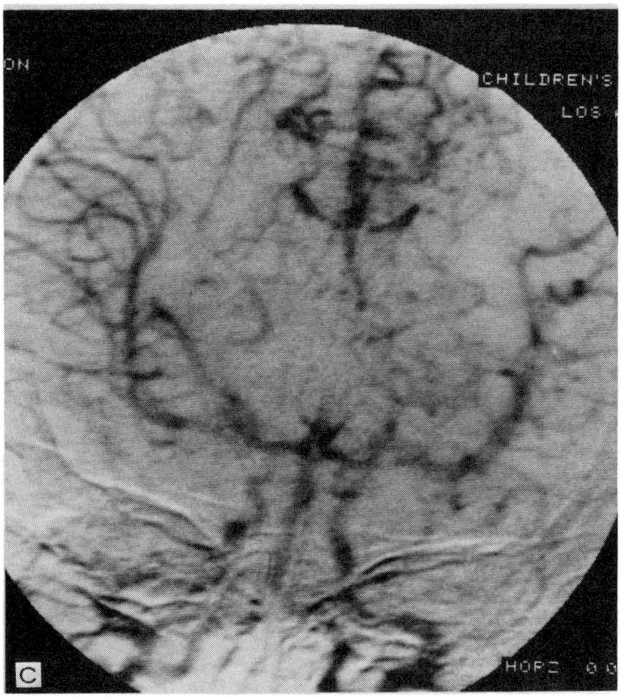

FIGURE 5C.

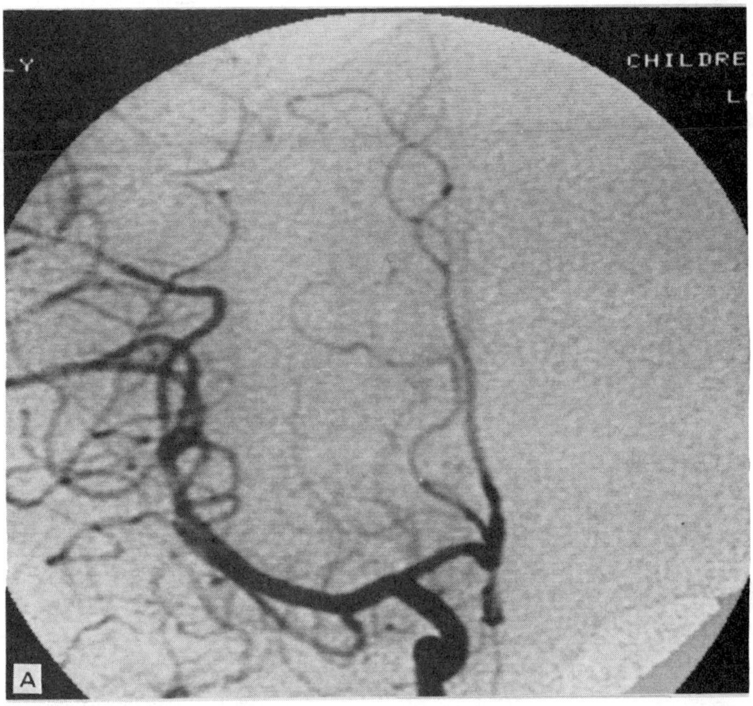

FIGURE 6A. Right carotid arteriogram showing excellent demonstration of the arterial anatomy. No abnormality was seen.

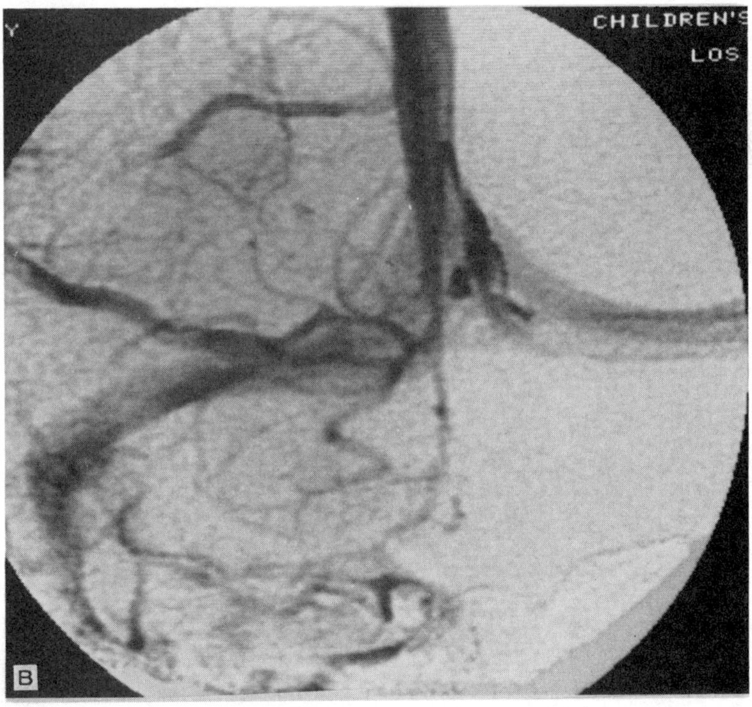

FIGURE 6B. Same patient; venous phase showing good visualization of the venous structures.

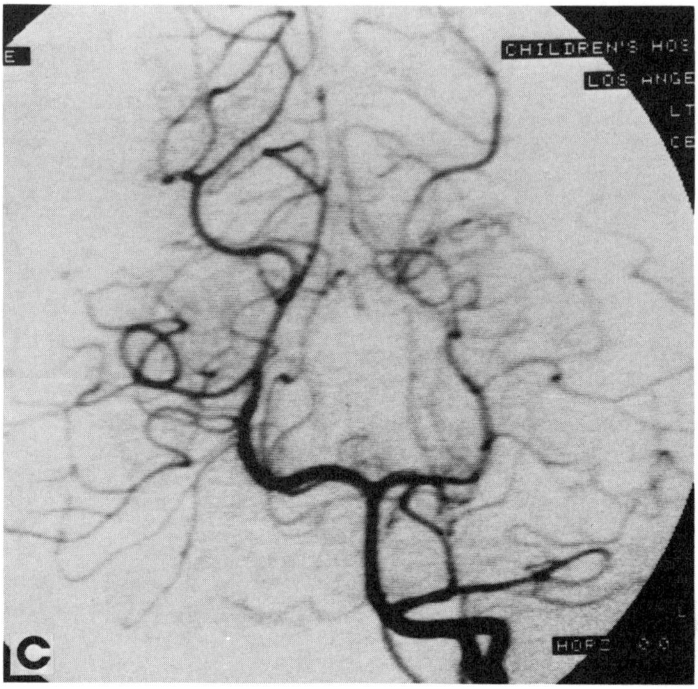

FIGURE 6C. Same patient; selective left vertebral arteriogram demonstrating excellent visualization of the arterial anatomy.

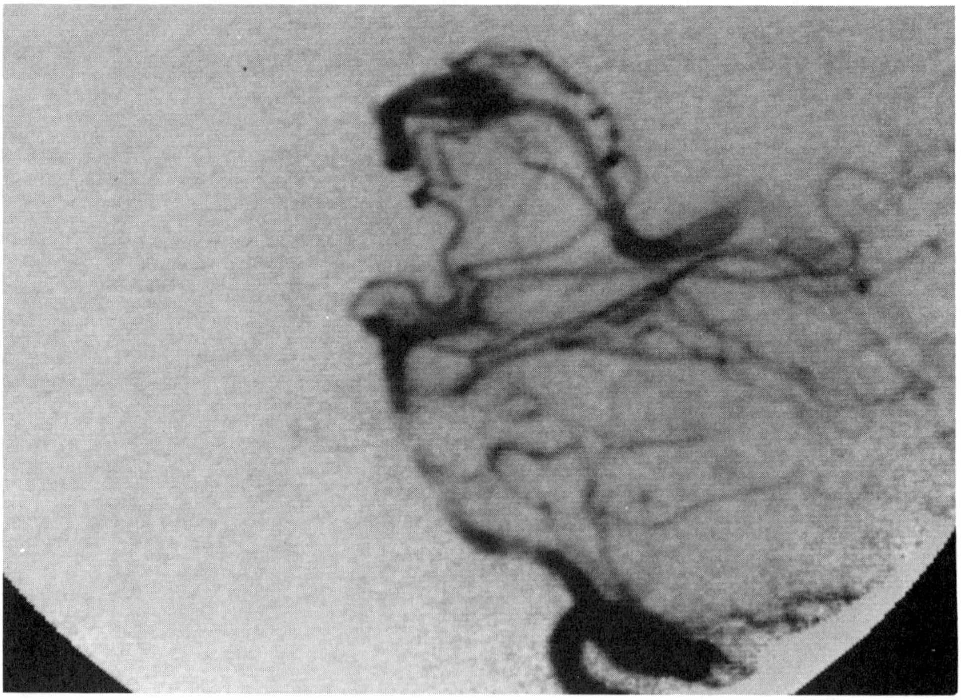

FIGURE 7. Lateral view of left vertebral arteriogram showing a thalamic arteriovenous malformation with supply from the posterior choroidal arteries.

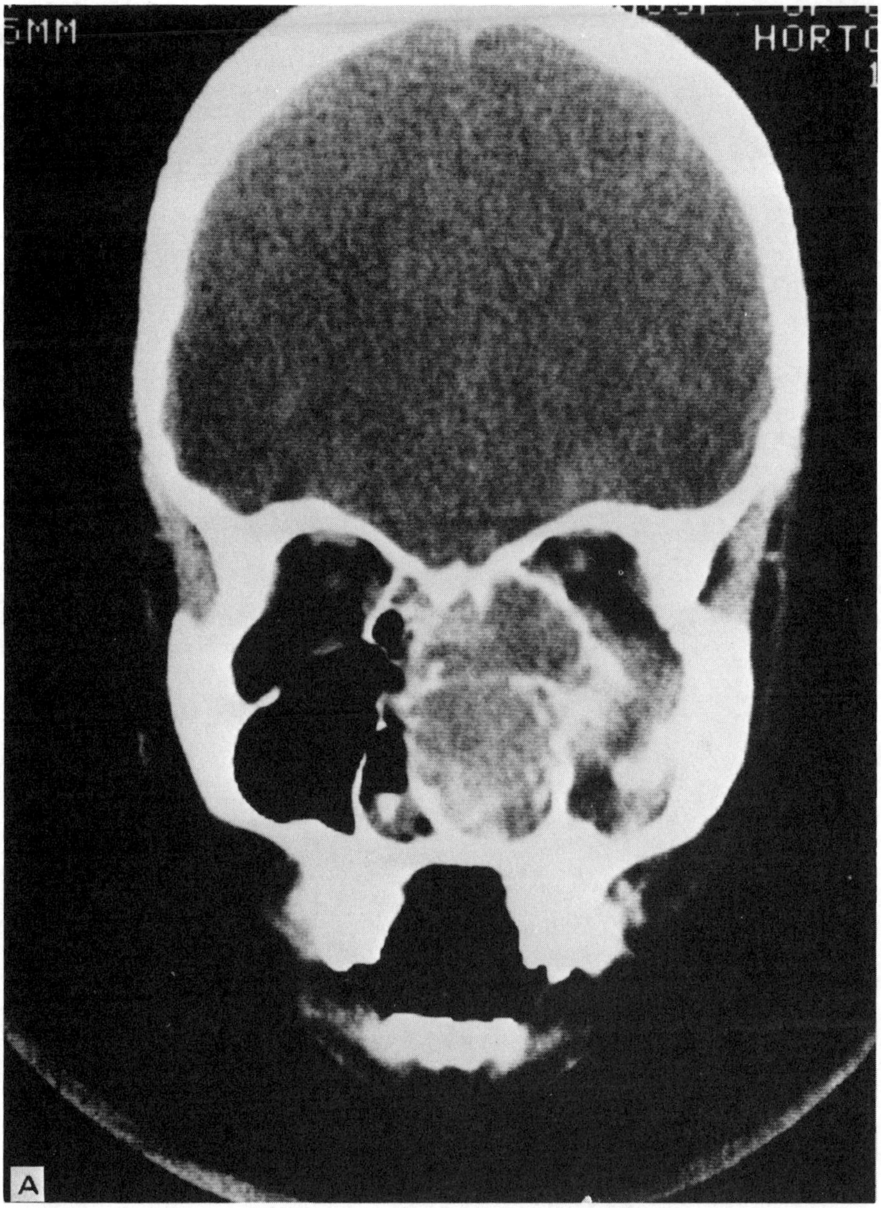

FIGURE 8. **A**: *Coronal CT showing a mass expanding and occupying the sphenoid sinus and posterior nares on the left with extension into the left antrum;* **B**: *Selective left external carotid arteriogram showing a hypertrophied internal maxillary artery with pathological circulation in the region of the tumor;* **C**: *Later phase demonstrates a hypervascular tumor in the region of the sphenoid sinus. These are the appearances of a juvenile nasal angiofibroma.*

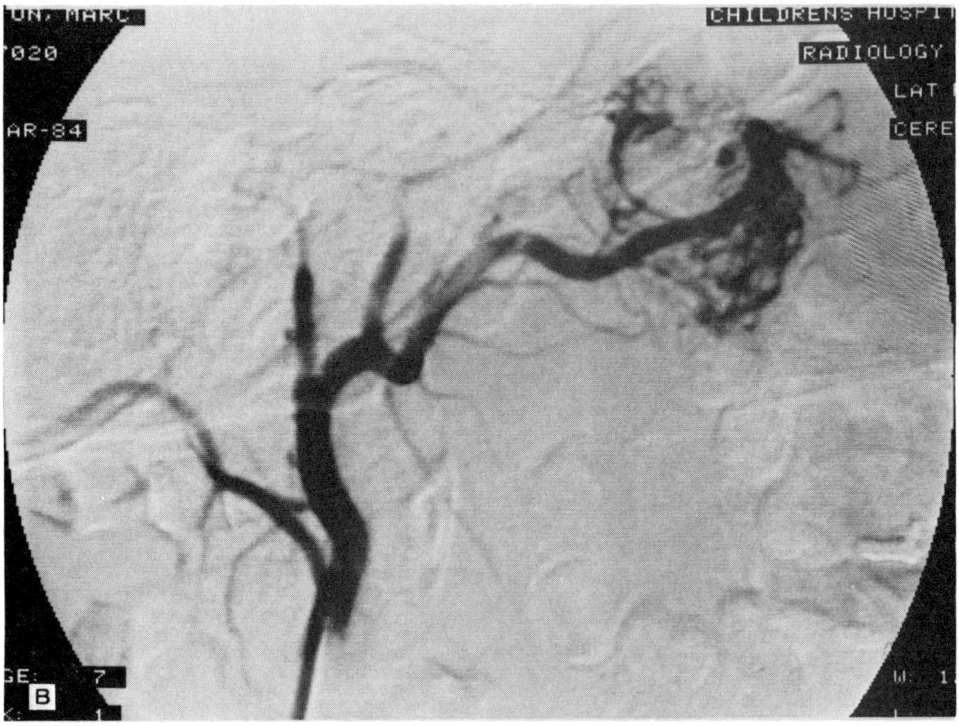

Figure 8B.

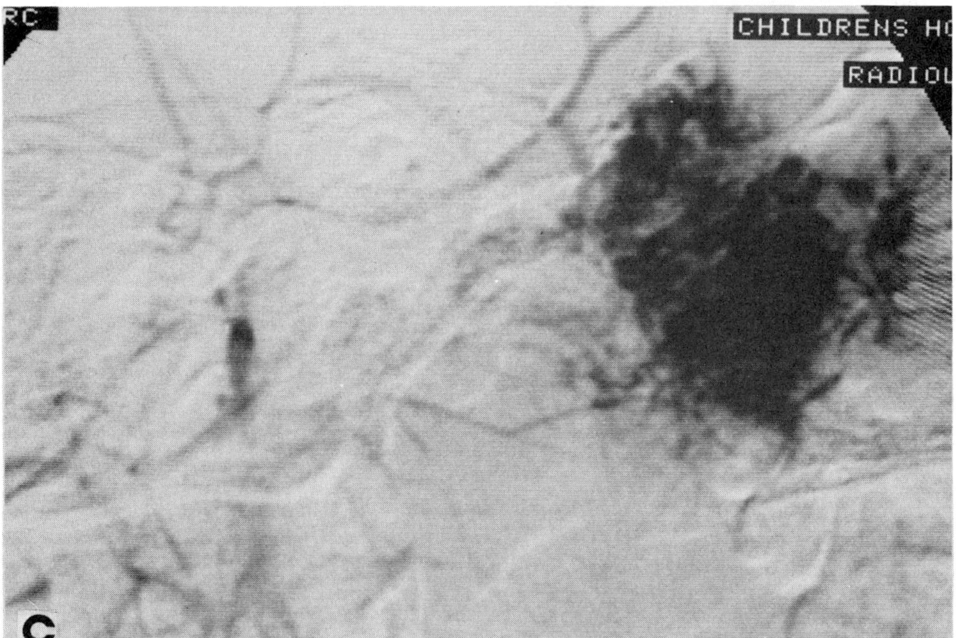

Figure 8C.

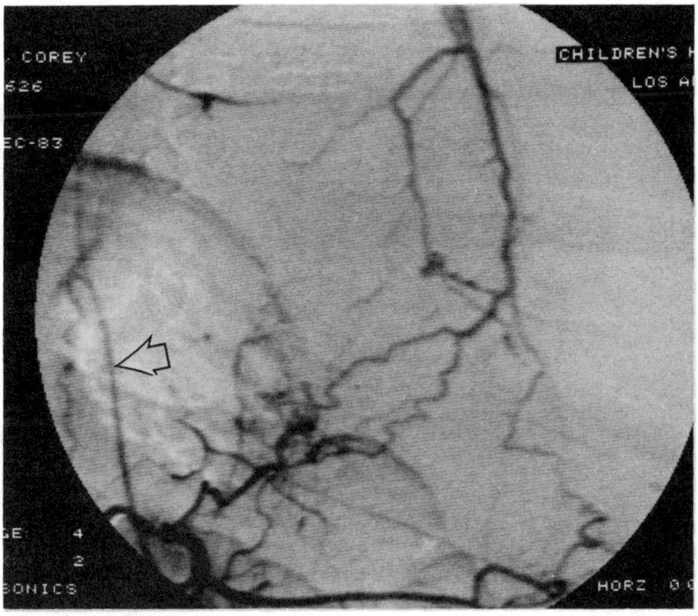

FIGURE 9. Intercostal arteriogram demonstrating pathologic circulation within a neuroblastoma. In addition, the artery of Adamkiewicz is also shown (open arrow). Embolization, although planned, was not performed because of the danger of occluding the anterior spinal artery.

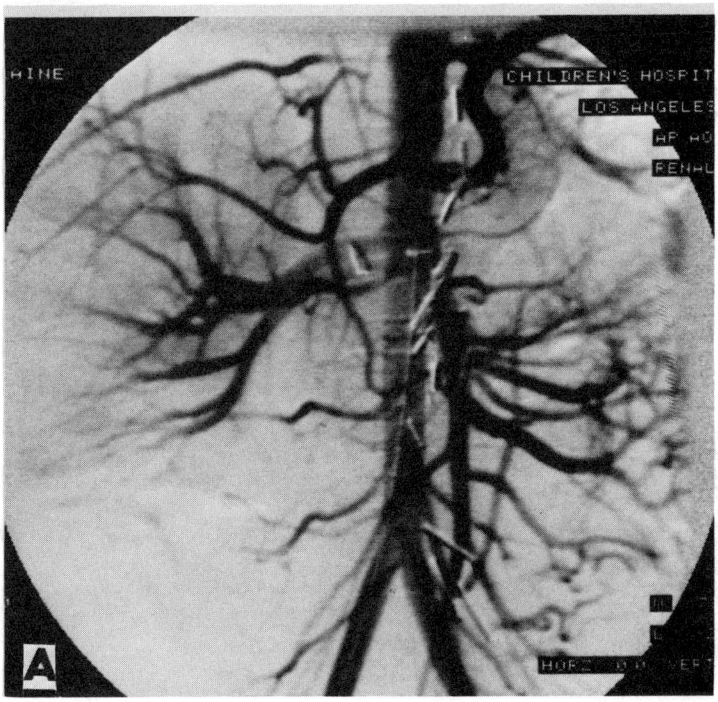

FIGURE 10A. Midstream aortogram performed in a girl with bilateral Wilms' tumors. The midstream aortogram was performed using a dilator.

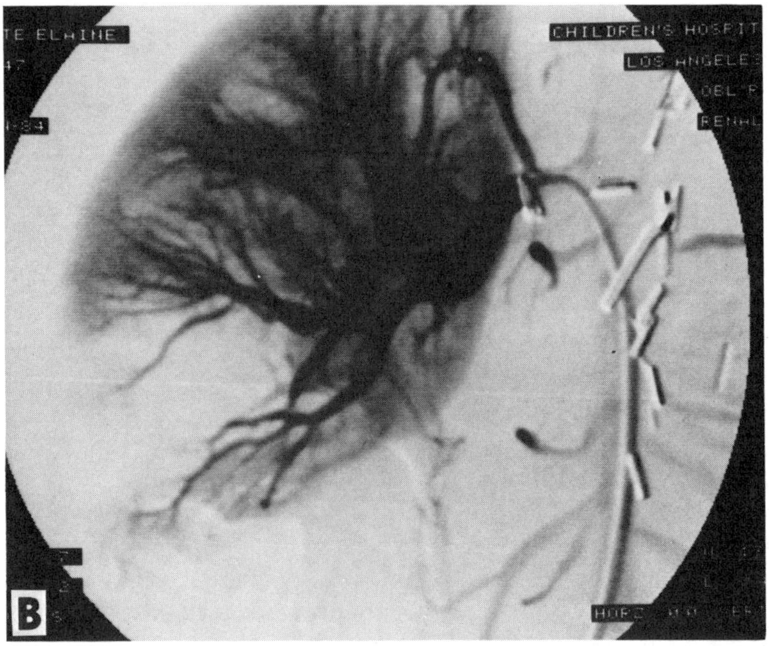

Figure 10B. Selective injection of the right kidney. The superior artery supplies most of the kidney.

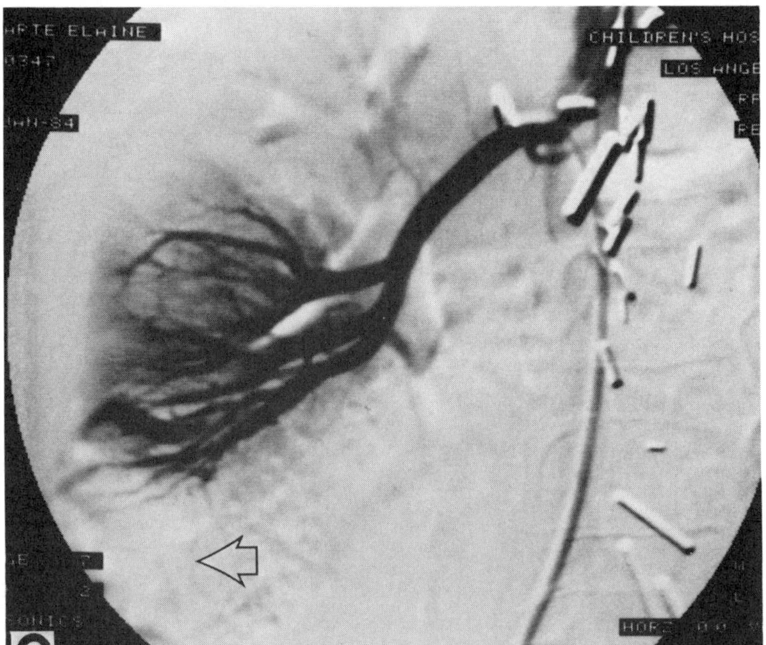

Figure 10C. Selective injection of the lower pole artery shows that there is subtle tumor vascularity (open arrow). This supplied a tumor arising from the lower pole.

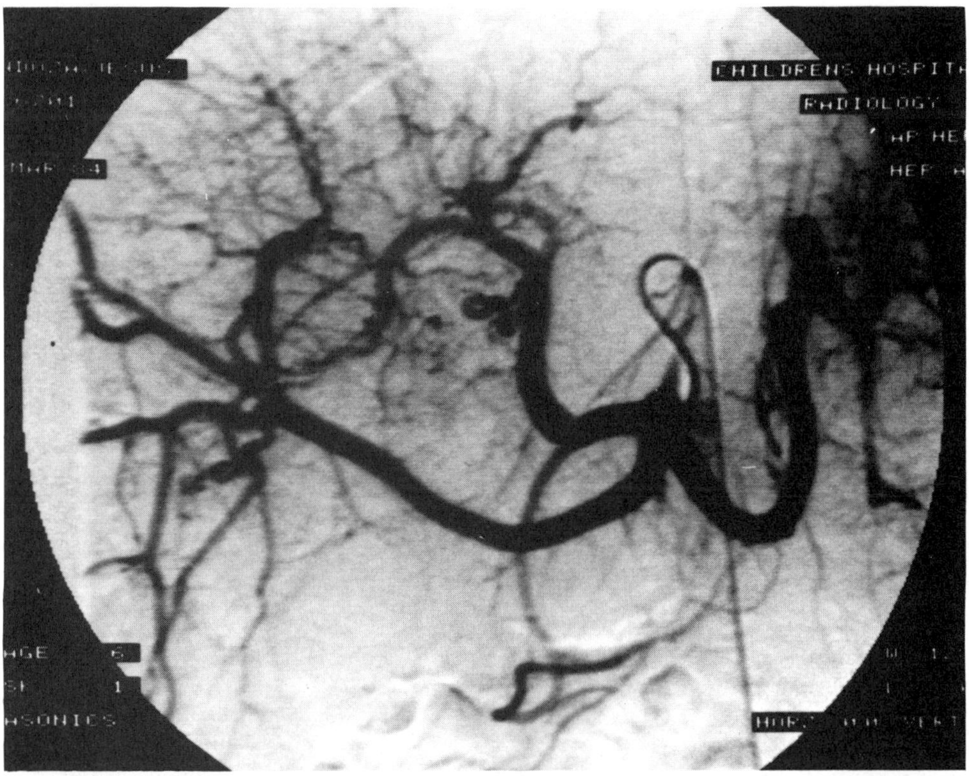

FIGURE 11. *Selective celiac axis arteriogram in a patient with a hepatic tumor. There is pathologic circulation arising from the left hepatic artery. The vascular anatomy was well demonstrated on this selective digital technique.*

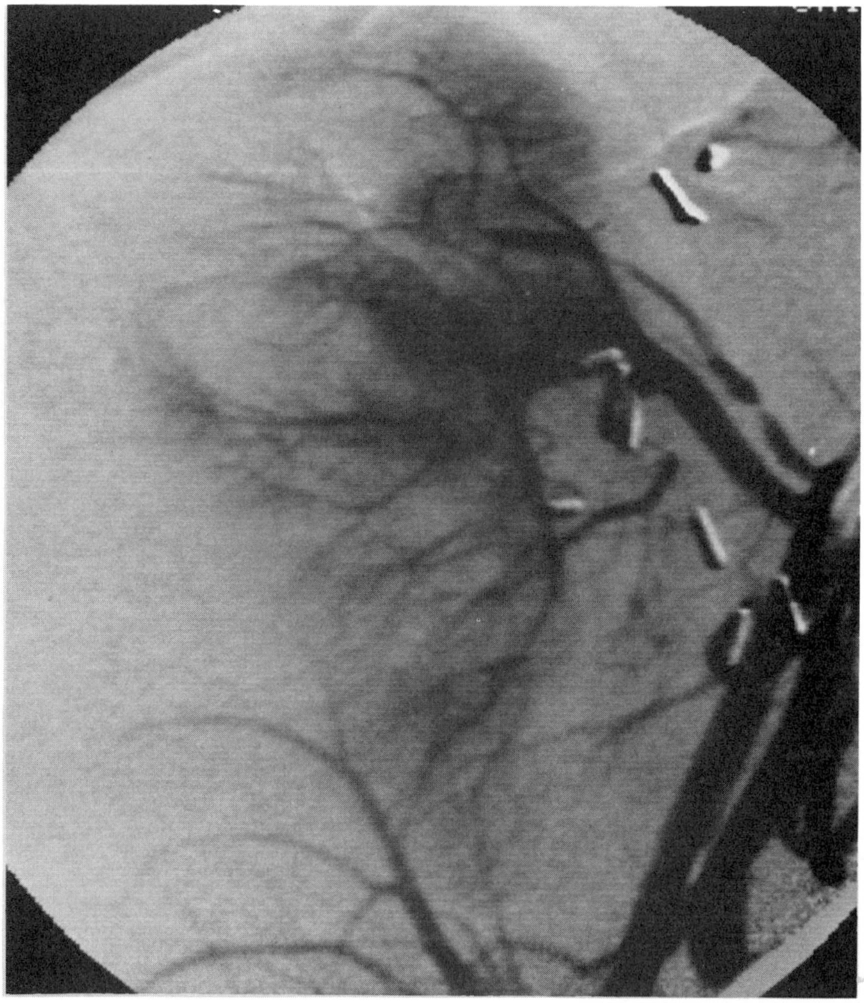

FIGURE 12. Transplant arteriogram performed with a dilator. There are two renal arteries to the transplant. There is marked irregularity of the superior and smaller artery. There are multiple defects within the kidney compatible with rejection.

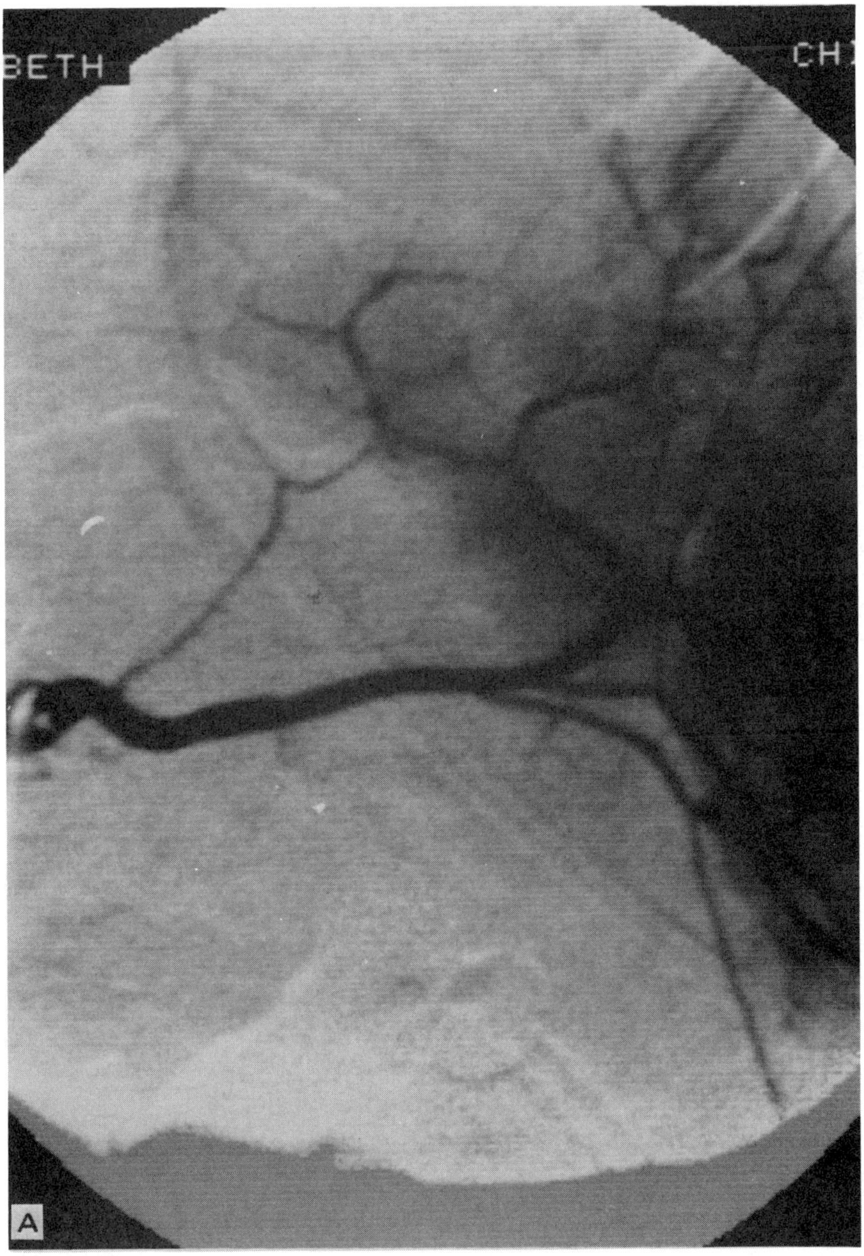

FIGURE 13A. Splenic arteriogram in a patient with portal hypertension and bleeding. There is slight irregularity of the splenic artery due to pancreatitis.

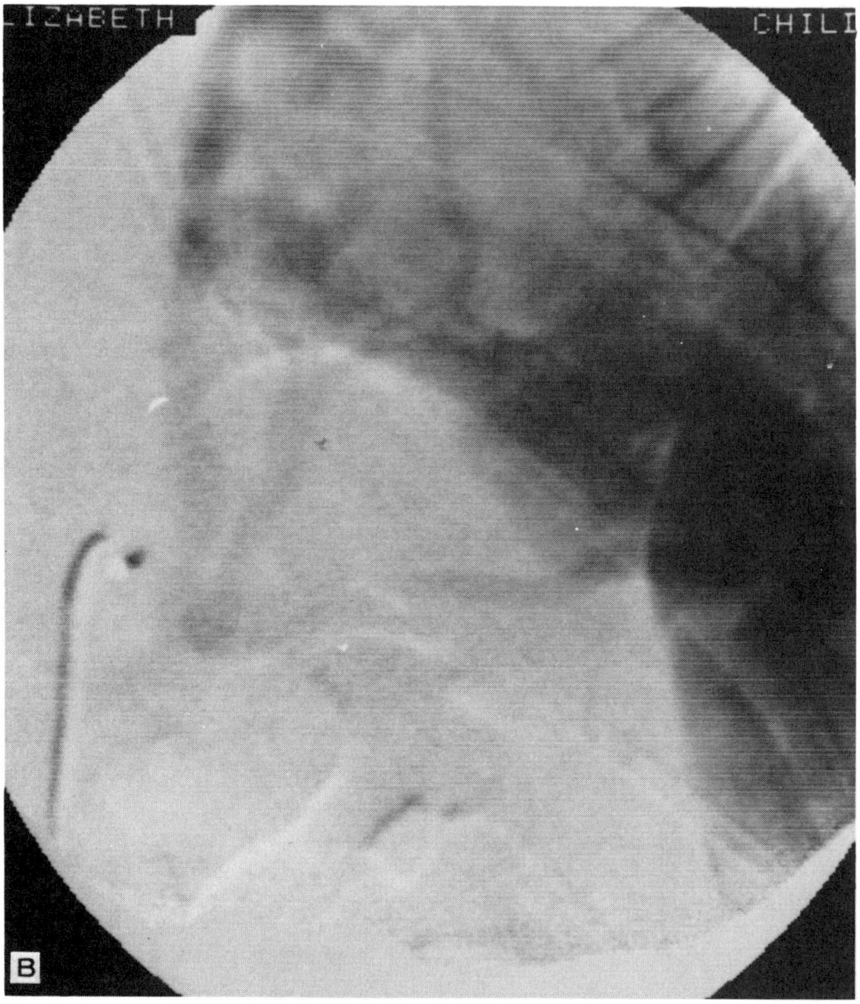

FIGURE 13B. Venous phase shows that the splenic vein has been thrombosed and is replaced by many collaterals. In addition, there were varices.

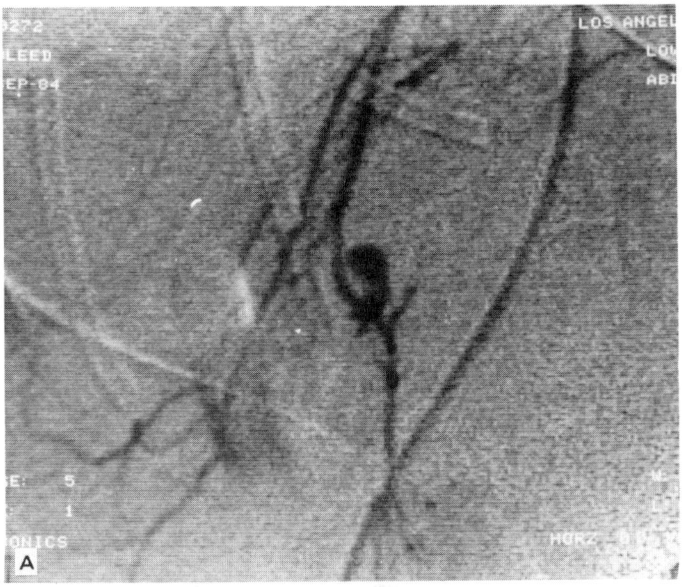

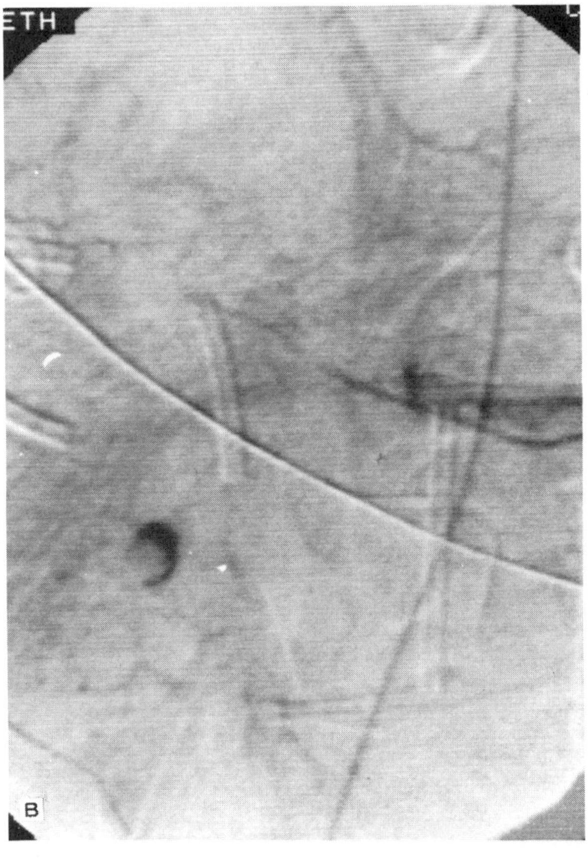

FIGURES 14A,B. Selective superior mesenteric arteriogram with placement of the catheter in an ileal branch. There is contrast extravasating from a small ileal artery. ***B****: Later phase shows contrast extravasating and retained within the bowel lumen.*

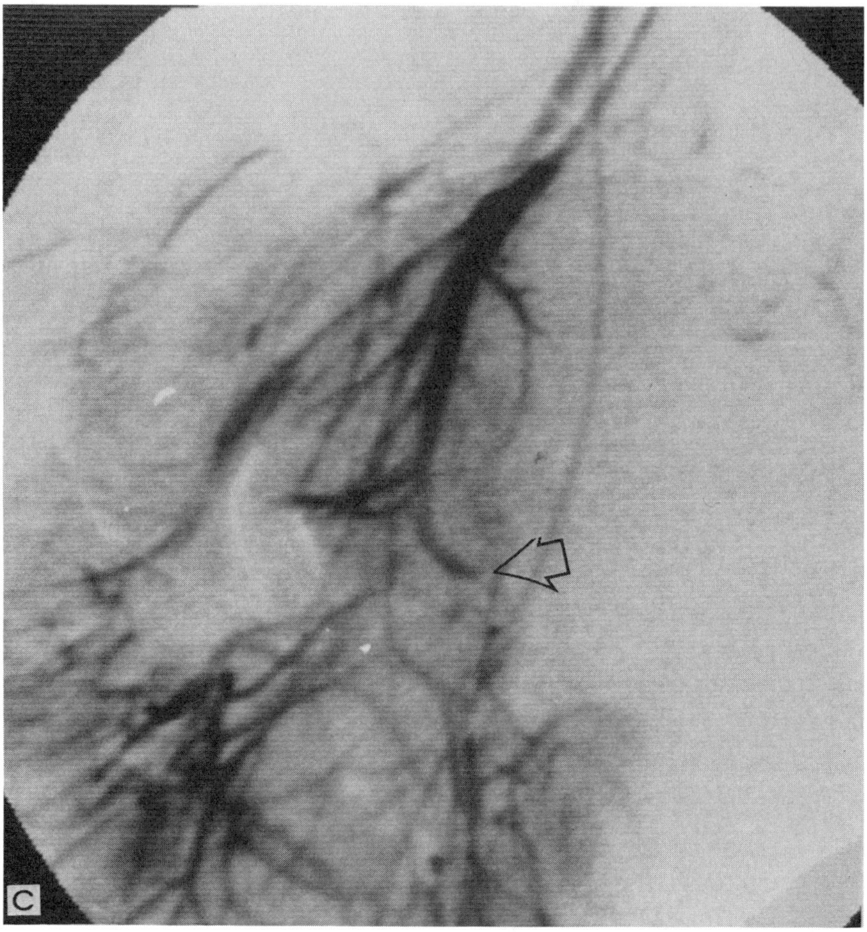

FIGURE 14C. Following therapeutic embolization, there is no evidence of bleeding. The occluded vessel is well demonstrated (open arrow).

duced.[6] Software refinements such as road mapping whereby the previous image is retained on the screen are particularly helpful. This aids catheter and guide wire manipulation in tortuous vessels. In addition, software programs will actually measure the dimension of a stenotic vessel, enabling the dilating balloon diameter to be accurately selected. Also, a satisfactory postdilatation angiogram may be obtained digitally by injecting contrast through the small lumen of the dilating catheter, which eliminates the need for catheter exchange. In children receiving local tumor chemotherapy, the position of the tip of the small caliber infusion catheter can be seen digitally, preventing inadvertent infusion of the wrong vessel.

References

1. Tonkin ILD, Gold RE, Moser D, Laster RE Jr: Evaluation of vascular rings with digital subtraction angiography. *AJR* 142:1287–1291, 1984.
2. Stadnik TW, Kersschot EAJ, De Schepper AMAP: Intracranial tumors examined by intraarterial DSA: A comparative angiography study. *Radiology* 154:671–675, 1985.
3. Stanley P, Malekzadeh M, Diament MJ: Posttransplant renal artery stenosis: Angiographic study in 32 children. *AJR* 148:487–490, 1987.
4. Braun SD, Newman GE, Dunnick NR: Digital splenoportography. *AJR* 144:1003–1004, 1985.
5. Zajko AB, Bron KM, Starzl TE, et al: Angiography of liver transplantation patients. *Radiology* 157:305–311, 1985.
6. Chang R, Kaufman SL, Kadir S, Mitchell SE, White RI Jr: Digital subtraction angiography in interventional radiology. *AJR* 142:363–366, 1984.

Chapter 4

Digital Subtraction Angiocardiography

Marie A. Capitanio, Richard M. Donner, and James N. Rauch

Introduction

Congenital heart disease is one of the most significant maladies affecting infants and young children. Of every 1,000 live births, 3.2 to 7.6 babies will have a congenital heart defect.[1] If these infants are not properly diagnosed and treated, more than 50% will die within the first year of life.[2,3] Conventional angiocardiography has long been one of the most important tools available for the diagnosis of congenital heart disease. Angiocardiography was first performed in children by Agustin Castellanos in 1936.[4] However, it was not until the introduction of the image-intensifier cinecamera to angiocardiography in the 1950s that angiocardiography in infants and children was routinely performed.[5] For more than forty years, conventional angiocardiography remained the single most reliable imaging tool for the assessment of the structure and function of the cardiovascular system.

The technologic advancements in the past 10 to 15 years have led to a greatly expanded approach to the diagnosis and treatment of congenital heart disease. Noninvasive or less invasive imaging modalities are now available by which the anatomy and function of the cardiovascular system may be accurately evaluated. These include computer-assisted radionuclide cardiovascular studies, M-mode and two-dimensional (2-D) real-time echocardiography, computed tomography, and more recently digital subtraction angiography (DSA), Doppler techniques, and magnetic resonance imaging.[6–11] Conventional angiocardiography continues to be the "gold standard" to which all the newer modalities are compared.

Digital Subtraction Imaging in Infants and Children, edited by Eric N. Faerber. Mount Kisco, New York: Futura Publishing Company, Inc., © 1989.

The purpose of this chapter is to review the current applications of DSA in the evaluation of congenital heart disease, recognizing that its role is still evolving. It is not the intent of the authors to review the general concepts and principles of angiocardiography in the evaluation of congenital heart disease, since the presently established standards apply irregardless of the imaging modality utilized.

Digital Subtraction Angiography

The first experimental application of DSA in the evaluation of patients with congenital heart disease occurred in the late 1970s.[12] It was not until 1980–81, however, that equipment for computed digital imaging became commercially available. This explains why abstract reports related to its clinical use in the evaluation of congenital heart disease did not appear in the literature until 1982.[13–16] The relative paucity of published papers on the use of DSA in the evaluation of congenital heart disease in infants and children since that time may be due to two major factors: (1) pediatric institutions, where large numbers of children with congenital heart disease are studied and treated, may not have digital equipment available; and (2) the role of less invasive modalities in the screening and diagnosis of congenital cardiovascular abnormalities is increasing.

The technical and physical aspects of digital radiography are presented in depth in Chapter 1; some of the technical factors that are of importance to digital subtraction angiocardiography will be briefly discussed here.

The *frame rate* requirements for digital subtraction imaging of the heart are considered to be greater than those for DSA of peripheral vessels or even the great vessels. Because of the motion of the heart, a frame rate of 30 frames/sec may be required and particularly if a cardiac functional analysis is desired.[18,19] On the other hand, the depiction of thoracic aortic anomalies in children has been achieved with a frame rate of 2 to 4/sec. For the evaluation of cardiac anatomy it has been suggested that the framing rate should be 8 or more frames/sec, however we have achieved diagnostic studies using only 3 frames/sec. When it is possible to use slower frame rates, such as 3 frames/sec, resolution is increased and the images can be directly digitized. Depending on the type of system used, images recorded at faster frame rates may not be directly digitized, but first must be recorded on disk or videotape in analog form and then converted to digital form by computer post processing.

The *site and method of injection* in cardiac DSA is of importance. Peripheral venous injections play little if any role in digital subtraction angiocardiography (IVDSA) in children. In instances of peripheral IVDSA, a relatively large bolus of contrast medium must be delivered rapidly. The veins of infants and young children are small and do not always permit the introduction of sufficiently large needles or catheters to deliver the required bolus.[20,21] For this reason, most IVDSA in infants is performed using a central vein such as the inferior vena cava or right atrium. In addition, to obtain optimal images more contrast medium is necessary using a peripheral vein than if central or selective intracardiac injections are made.[22]

With selective intracardiac injections the concentration and volume of contrast medium for DSA can be decreased by 50%.[23–25] This is of great significance as the amount of contrast medium that can be used in infants and small children is often a limiting factor. Since angiocardiography in infants and children is most often performed at the time of cardiac catheterization (a necessary procedure to obtain pressure and oxygen saturation measurements), selective intracardiac injections can be readily carried out. It should be noted that nonionic as well as standard ionic contrast agents can be used in both DSA as well as in conventional angiocardiographic studies in children.

There is virtually no role for the use of IVDSA in the evaluation of children with complex cardiac anomalies or in instances of multilevel shunting. In addition, IVDSA is of little value in the evaluation of newborns suspected of having right-to-left shunting as may occur in the presence of a congenital heart defect or persistent fetal circulation. If significant right-to-left shunting is occurring, the amount of contrast medium that returns to the left side of the heart will be small when IVDSA is performed and will result in poor quality images of the pulmonary venous return and the left side of the heart.[18] IVDSA has been of value in the evaluation of abnormalities of the aorta such as coarctation of the aorta and vascular rings[26,27] which are discussed in Chapter 5.

Visualization of the hypoplastic aorta in the hypoplastic left heart syndrome may be achieved by injecting the contrast medium into the right brachial artery. The forward arterial blood flow in this syndrome is decreased and retrograde opacification of the ascending aorta is readily accomplished (Fig. 1).

The *acquisition and processing* of fluoroscopic data for cardiac imaging have been well discussed in the scientific literature.[16,19,28–35] In general, the video signals may be directly digitized and immediately processed or the video signals may be recorded on videotape and later digitized with post processing of the images with the computer. Following computer processing (subtraction, filtering, etc.) the digital data can be reversed to an analog form for display on a video monitor or in a film format. Although the technique of postprocessing results in the introduction of some noise, adequate images of the chambers of the heart, which are relatively large, can be obtained. To achieve visualization of smaller and relatively stationary peripheral arteries with high resolution, therefore, direct digitization of the amplified video signal may be essential.

As a rule, useful information from a digital study using the postprocessing method will depend on the method used for masking. The masking procedure entails finding a frame or frames in which there is no contrast medium present and that best match(es) the background of a frame or frames in which the structures to be evaluated are opacified. There are two basic problems encountered in the masking process. One occurs if the contrast medium becomes too dilute at the time it reaches the area of interest. The dilution of the contrast medium can be a significant factor when peripheral venous sites are used for injection or, similarly, if the site of injection is the right side of the heart when attempting to evaluate pulmonary venous return.

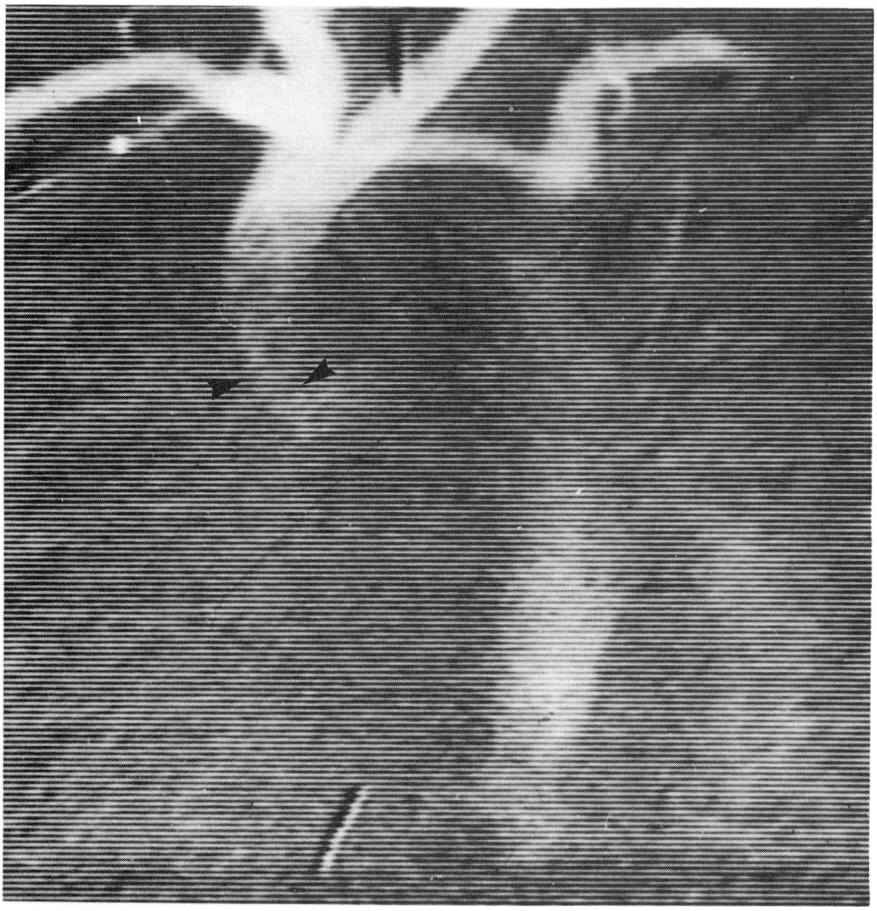

FIGURE 1. The hypoplastic ascending aorta (arrowheads) of an infant with hypoplastic left heart syndrome was demonstrated by injecting contrast medium into the right brachial artery.

The other major factor that interferes with the masking process is patient motion, including respiratory and cardiac motion. To minimize these difficulties and achieve successful masking, several measures should be taken during the course of the study.

First, to ensure adequate opacification the amount, concentration, and flow rate of the contrast agent to be injected should be carefully selected; the site of the injection and the region of interest to be studied will be determining factors. It is important to note, that using too much contrast medium can result in an image with poor definition, as well as being potentially injurious to the child.

Second, to minimize motion the child should be appropriately sedated and immobilized. The cooperative child is instructed to hold his breath in order to minimize respiratory motion while the data are being recorded. The use of ECG-gating and short pulse width will reduce the masking difficulties produced by cardiac motion and result in high quality images.

Third, the field should be magnified as much as possible, making certain that the region(s) of interest can be viewed.

Fourth, the frame rate to be used depends on how fast the contrast medium flows through the area of interest. As a rule, slower frame rates will yield better resolution but with higher radiation output per frame than faster frame rates.

Another important process that can be used in DSA to suppress motion artifacts and achieve optimal images is remasking. In remasking, the original images are reviewed and two are selected to make a remasked image. The selection of the images is usually a trial and error process. Generally, using the image immediately preceding the arrival of the bolus and the image with peak contrast will result in the best remasked image.

Pixel shifting is another technique used in DSA to remove motion artifacts. The mask and contrast-filled images are electronically shifted with respect to each other prior to subtraction in order to register the mobile structure in the two images.

Cardiac Anatomy

The application of DSA for the evaluation of congenital cardiovascular anomalies since its introduction in the early 1980s would appear to be increasing, as evidenced by the number of reports in the literature since the first abstracts[13–16] appeared in 1982. Most of the papers published to date have been concerned with the use of IVDSA in children.[5,6,18,24,35–41] Although there has been limited experience in the use of intra-arterial digital subtraction angiography (IADSA) in children, Tonkin and others have suggested that, in the future, IADSA and intracardiac DSA may replace conventional film/screen angiography and cineangiography in children.[36,42–44]

In the early applications of IVDSA in the evaluation of congenital heart disease (CHD) the conventional anteroposterior and lateral or right and left anterior oblique projections were utilized. It is now recognized that the axial projection is far superior to the previous conventional views in defining the cardiac anatomy.[45] By means of the "four-chamber view," there is less superimposition of the left and right atria and ventricles. In addition, this view exposes more of the ventricular septum thus allowing for better localization of ventricular septal defects. The four-chamber projection is suitable for IVDSA as well as for selective intracardiac DSA (Fig. 2).

Left-to-right shunting across an atrial or ventricular septal defect can be readily appreciated by means of IVDSA, although visualizing the actual ventricular septal defect(s), unless of moderate size, is somewhat more difficult than visualizing atrial septal defects. IVDSA has also proven to be of value in the evaluation of the adequacy of the surgical repair of septal defects.[46]

Many of the congenital anomalies of the systemic and pulmonary veins have been readily demonstrated by DSA as has the evaluation of the surgical repair of such anomalies. Other congenital defects have been satisfactorily visualized such as: patent ductus arteriosus, tricuspid atresia, Ebstein's anomaly,

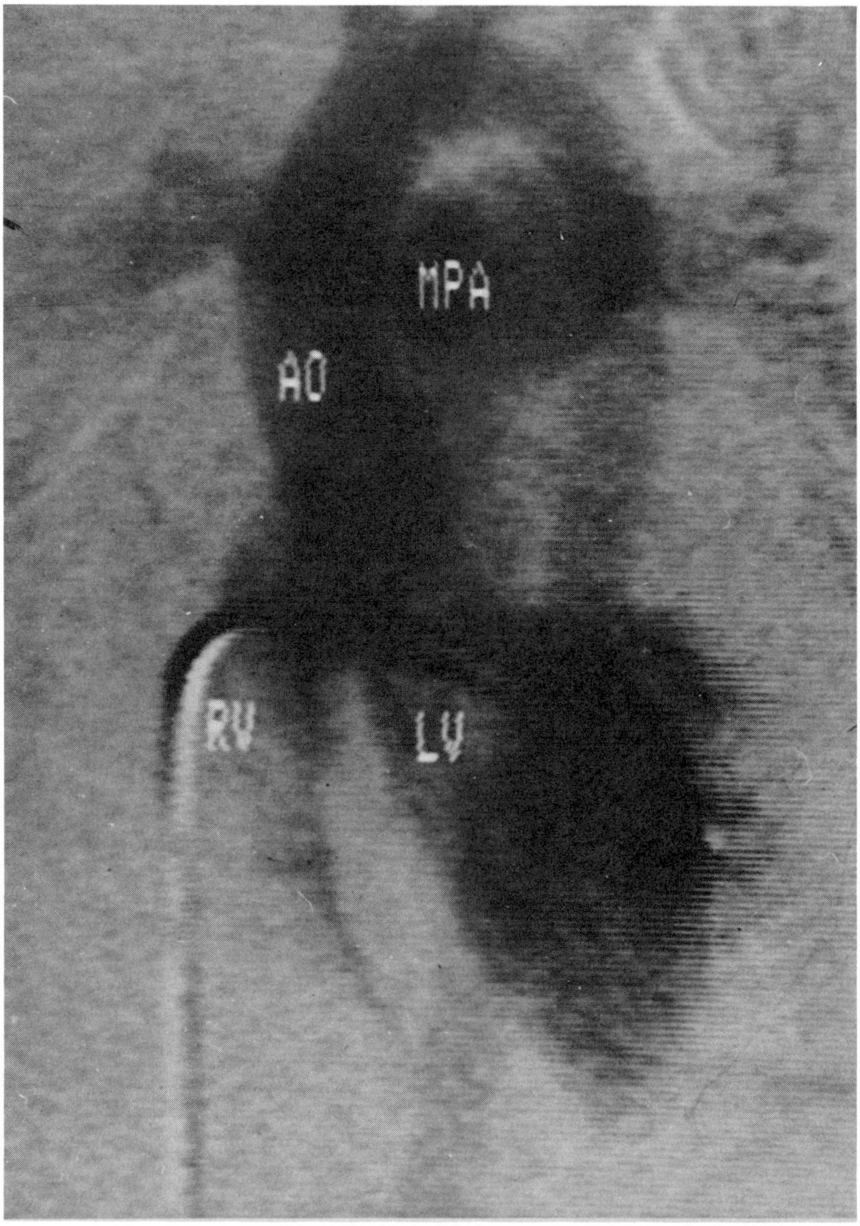

FIGURE 2. Note excellent visualization of the ventricular septum in the "four-chamber view" in this child with a VSD. (The injection was into the left ventricle via a catheter passed through the VSD). AO = aorta; RV = right ventricle; LV = left ventricle; MPA = main pulmonary artery.

transposition of the great vessels, tetralogy of Fallot, single ventricle, hypoplastic left heart, and other complex cardiac defects.[15,19,22,25,36–39,45] (Figs. 3–7).

The assessment of pre- and postoperative digital subtraction angiocardiograms in CHD has been reported by a number of authors.[42,46–48] In the preoperative studies of 13 patients with tetralogy of Fallot, Moodie was able to visualize the location of the VSD, overriding aorta, previous systemic pulmonary artery shunts, abnormalities of the outflow tract, and the closure of the ventricular septal defect (VSD) in all patients. The postoperative DSA studies demonstrated a small residual ventricular septal defect in 1 patient, outflow patch aneurysm in 2 patients, proximal right pulmonary artery stenosis in 1 patient, and in 2 patients a hypoplastic and distorted left pulmonary artery due to a previous shunt.[42]

Fifty-eight patients were studied by Vogel et al. in the immediate postoperative period by DSA.[46] Forty-five of their patients had a transposition of the great vessels and had had an atrial inversion with the Senning procedure. The confluence of the superior and inferior vena cavae into the systemic venous

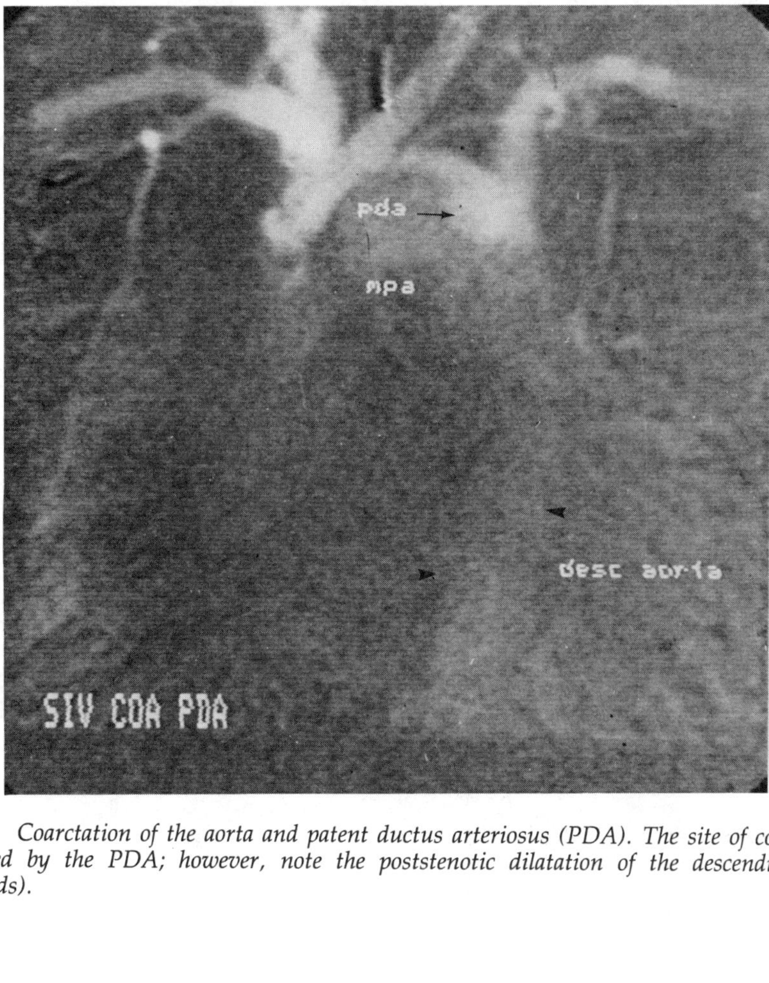

FIGURE 3. Coarctation of the aorta and patent ductus arteriosus (PDA). The site of coarctation is obscured by the PDA; however, note the poststenotic dilatation of the descending aorta (arrowheads).

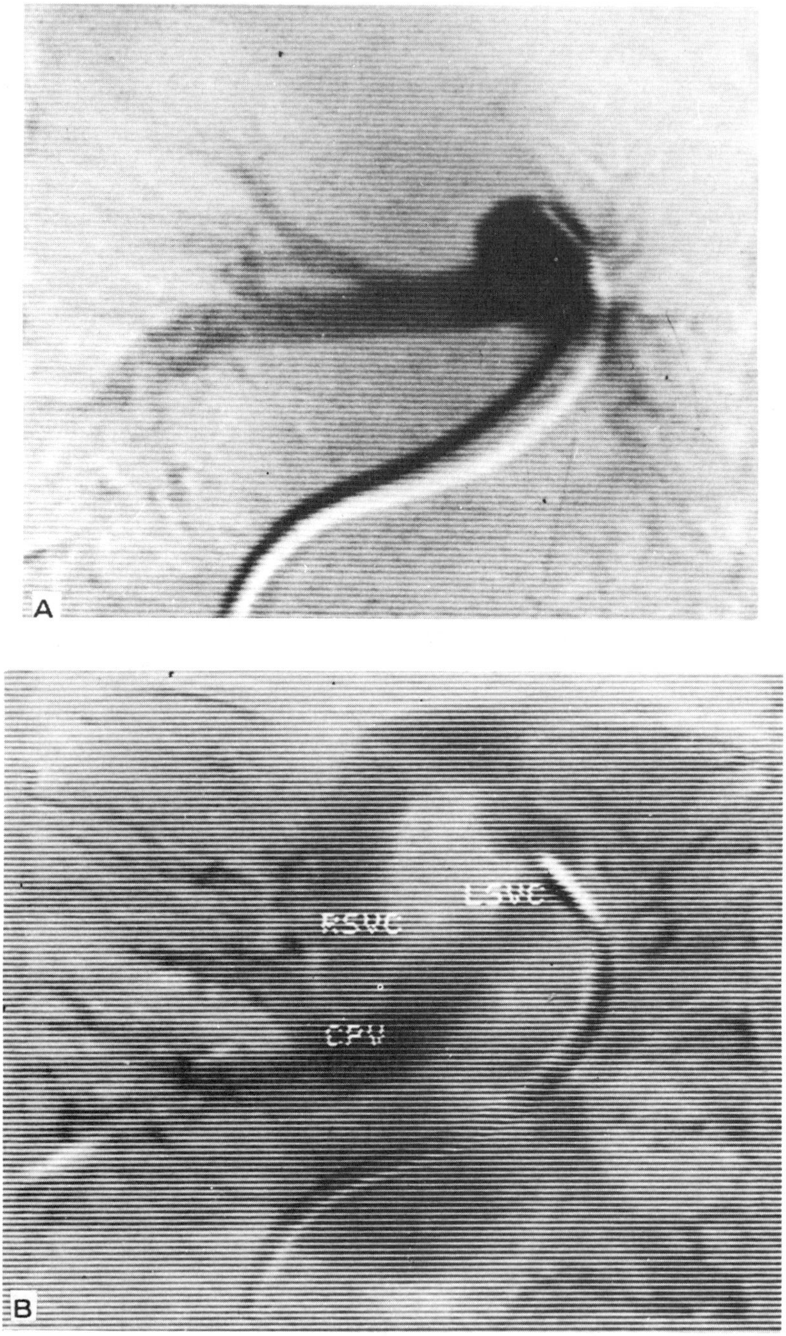

*FIGURE 4. Total anomalous pulmonary venous return (TAPVR). Contrast medium was injected into the main pulmonary artery (**A**) and recorded into the levophase (**B**) demonstrating the anomaly of the pulmonary veins. CPV = common pulmonary vein; LSVC = left superior vena cava; RSVC = right superior vena cava.*

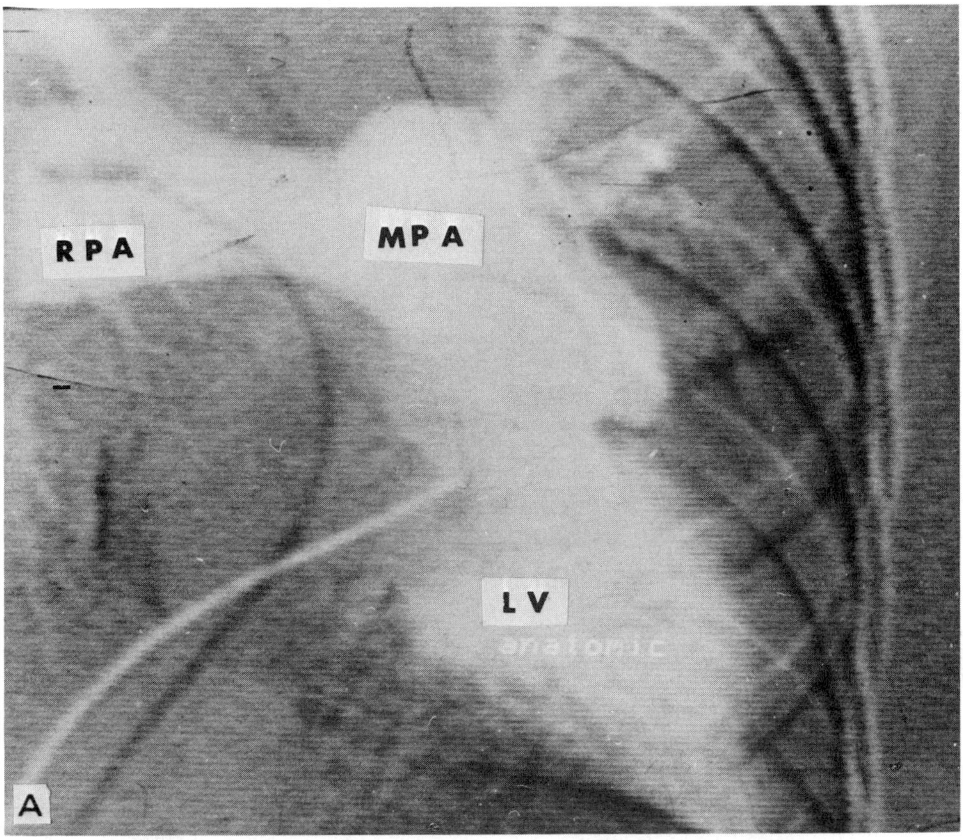

*FIGURE 5. Transposition of the great vessels (TGV). The catheter has been passed through a VSD from the right ventricle into the left ventricle where the injection of contrast medium was made. The main pulmonary artery arises from the left ventricle (**A**) and after pulmonary venous return to the left atrium with subsequent left-to-right shunting at the atrial level opacification of the right heart is demonstrated as is the origin of the aorta from the right ventricle (**B**). By means of computer manipulation a composite image was reconstructed (**C**). RPA = Right pulmonary artery; MPA = main pulmonary artery; LV = left ventricle.*

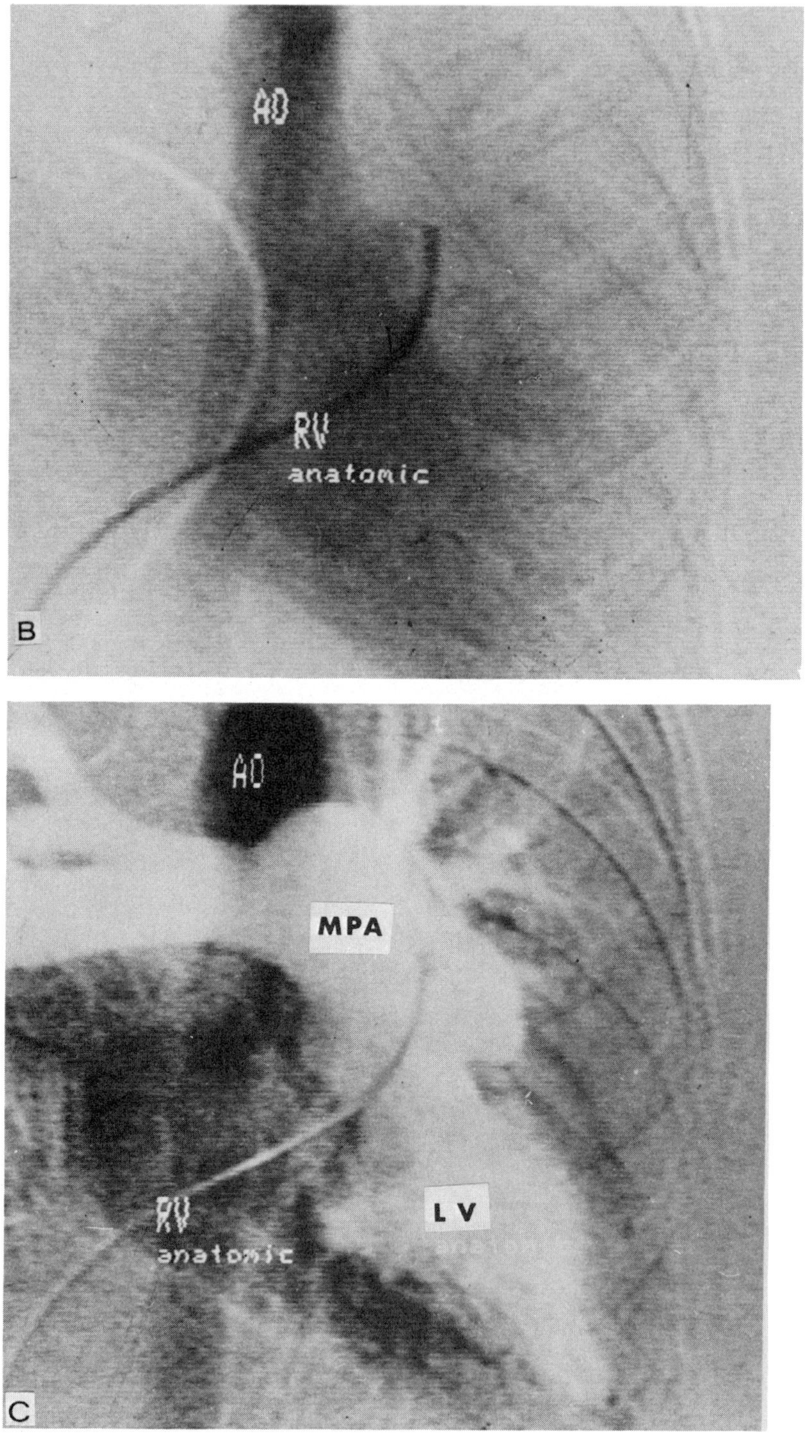

Figures 5B, C.

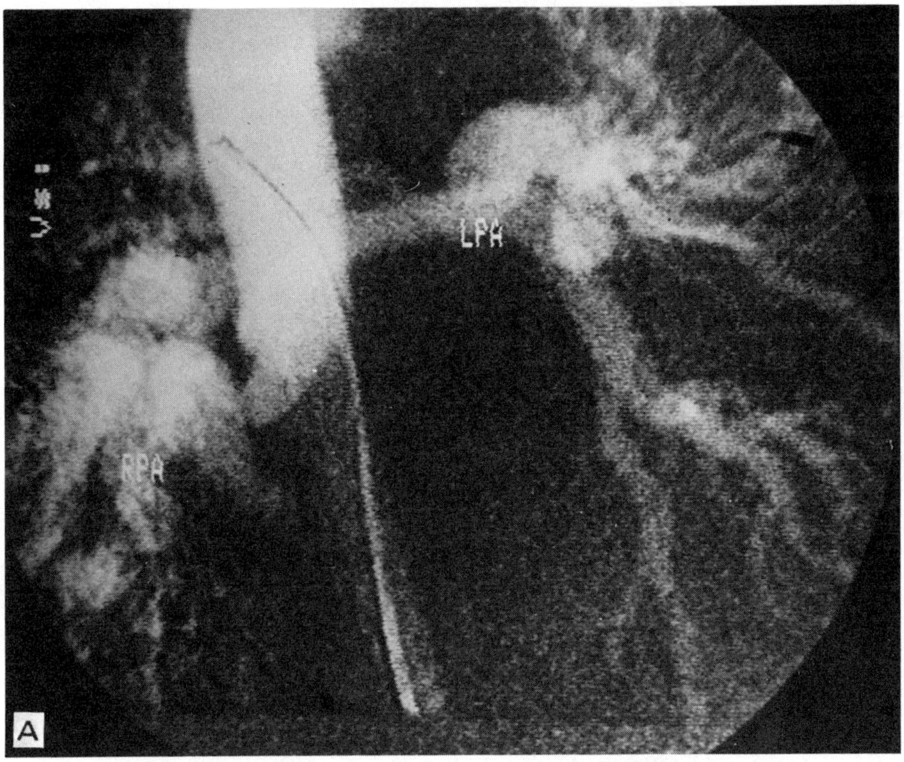

*FIGURE 6. Severe tetralogy of Fallot with pulmonary atresia. The flow to the lungs from aortic collaterals is well demonstrated by an injection of contrast medium into the descending aorta (**A**) as is the evaluation of pulmonary venous return and the left side of the heart (**B**). By means of a centimeter ruler (**C**) the size of the pulmonary arteries can be measured as demonstrated in (**D**) where the pulmonary arteries are well visualized following a selective injection into one of the collateral vessels arising from the aorta. This is especially important when planning shunt procedures to improve blood flow to the lungs. RPA = right pulmonary artery; LPA = left pulmonary artery; LUPV = left upper pulmonary artery; RUPV = right upper pulmonary artery; RMPV = right middle pulmonary artery; RLPV = right lower pulmonary artery.*

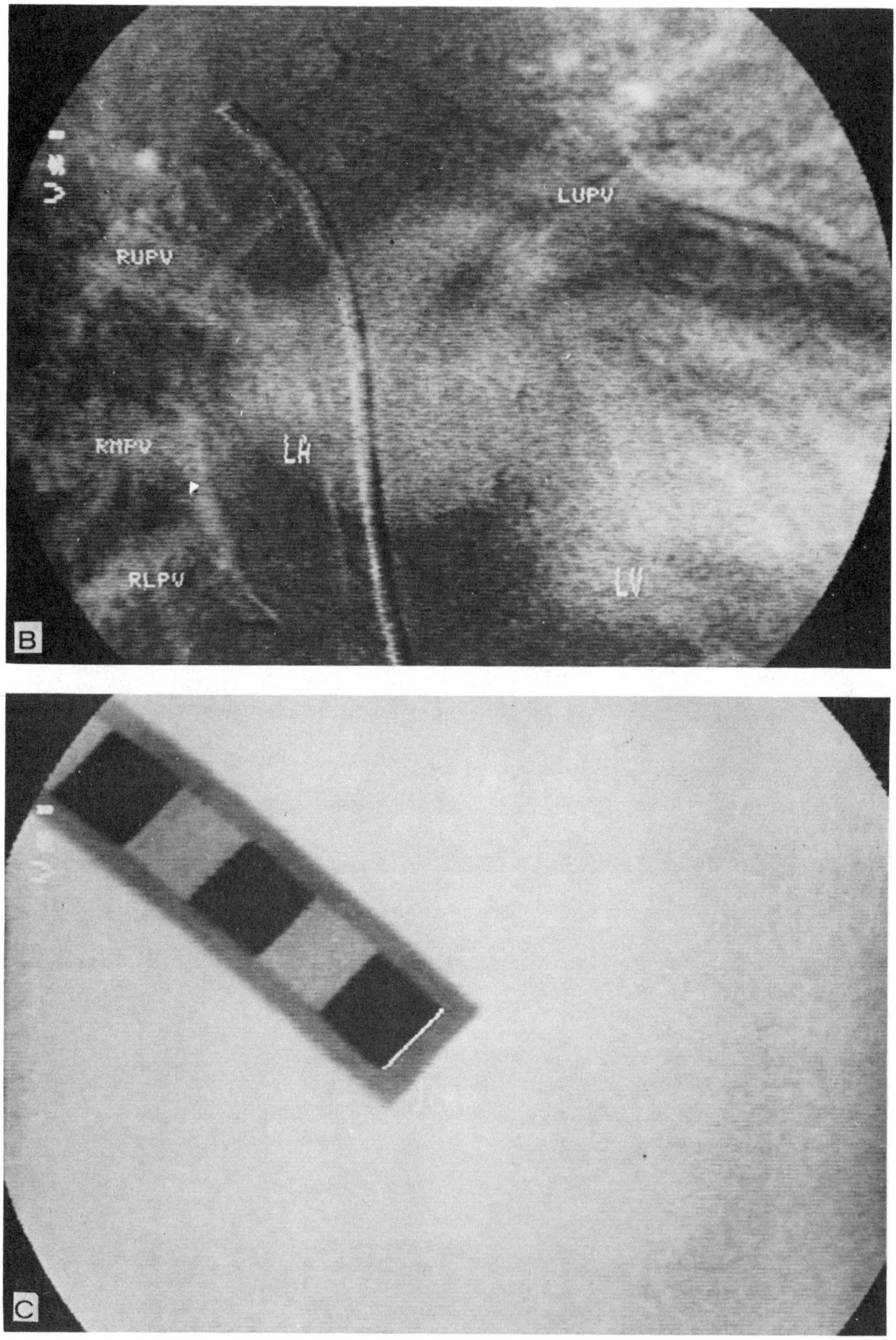

Figures 6B, C.

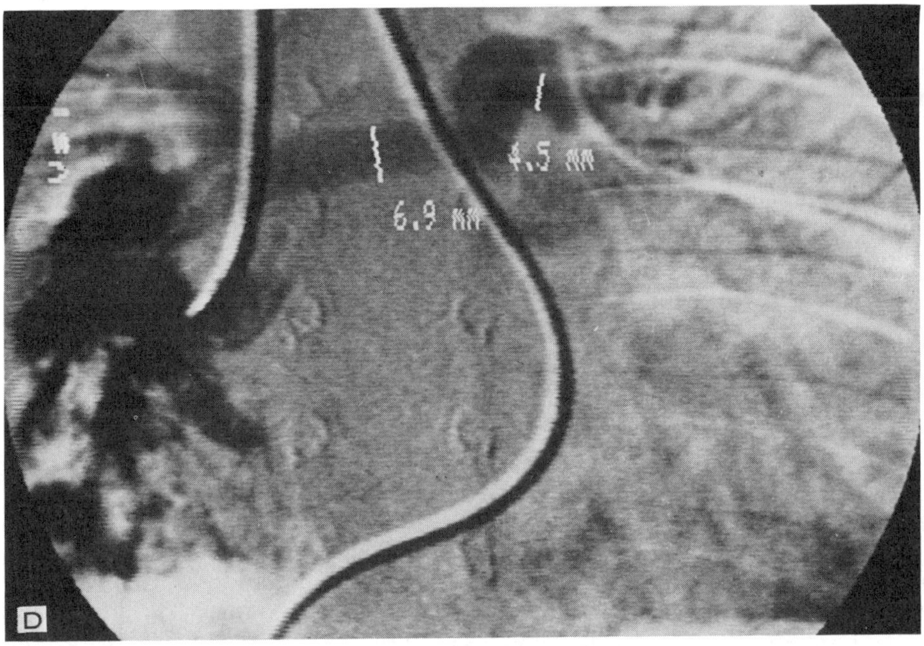

FIGURE 6D.

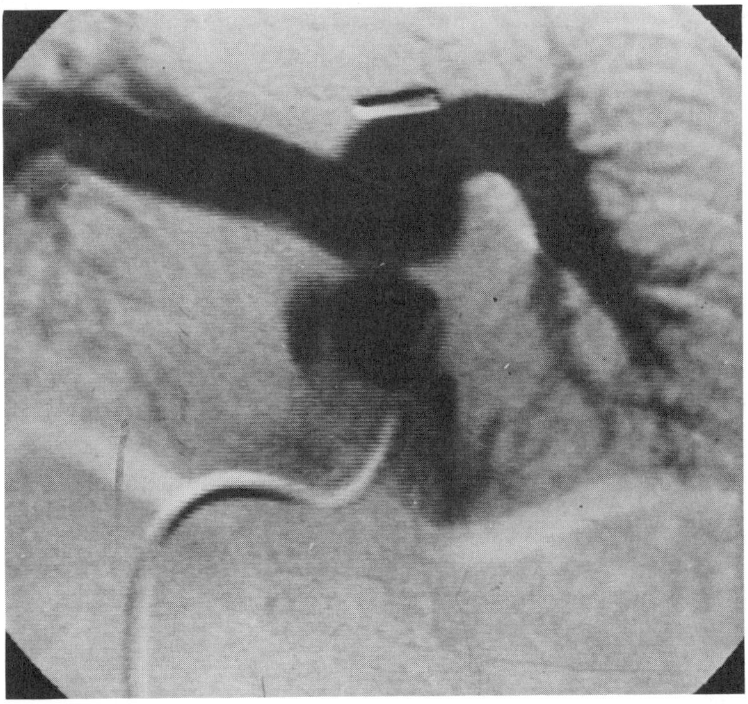

FIGURE 7. *Banding of main pulmonary artery. A digital subtraction pulmonary arteriogram affords excellent visualization of the constriction of the main pulmonary artery by a surgically placed band.*

portion of the atrium was demonstrated in all 45 patients and in one-third of the patients the pulmonary veins were visualized. An obstruction of the superior vena cavae as well as the collateral circulation via the azygos vein and the inferior vena cava was demonstrated in 8 patients.

Digital subtraction angiocardiography has been shown to be successful in demonstrating the precise diagnosis in more than 85% of patients with congenital heart defects.[49] In addition, tumors of the heart and abnormalities of the pulmonary arteries and of the coronary arteries have been successfully evaluated by DSA.[7,42,44]

Shunt Quantification

The quantification of the degree of left-to-right shunting is possible by means of digital subtraction angiocardiography. The calculation of pulmonary to systemic flow (Qp/Qs) ratios from the DSA study utilizes the technique that is applied to radionuclide studies. In the case of the DSA study, a videodensitometric cursor is placed on the pulmonary artery or a region of the heart. Flow curves can then be developed representing the appearance and clearance of contrast medium. By means of a gamma fit of the curves, the degree of shunting can be quantified.[12] The gamma fit of a curve is used in radionuclide studies to separate the activity caused by the first pulmonary transit from that of early recirculation due to a shunt.[50] This method applies readily to the calculation of Qp/Qs ratios from DSA studies. Moodie showed that the Qp/Qs ratios determined from DSA studies correlated well with the Qp/Qs ratios obtained from radionuclide studies ($r = 0.89$) in 25 patients who had shunts documented and quantified by cardiac catheterization.[42,47,48]

Functional Analysis

The use of DSA in the evaluation of cardiac function has been performed primarily for the assessment of left ventricular function in patients with acquired heart disease. Methods have been developed whereby the dimensions of the left ventricle can be ascertained, the left ventricular ejection fraction and cardiac output can be measured, and the wall motion of the left ventricle demonstrated.[18,51–54]

Functional studies using DSA are possible because digital imaging systems provide real-time acquisition of data with rates up to 30 frames/sec. This is of importance for flow studies of the central circulation in which high imaging rates are needed to resolve temporal changes in image contrast. Conversely, rates as low as 4 frames/sec can be used for functional studies of the peripheral circulation where the flow rate is considerably slower. Whenever possible, however, it is best to use low frame rates. The real-time storage capacity of some digital systems is limited and a significant amount of data may not be recorded if increased frame rates are utilized. In such instances, when fast frame rates are used, large numbers of frames will need to be processed which will prolong the processing time significantly.[51]

Functional analysis by means of current digital systems is feasible because such systems permit the outlining of regions of interest and the recording of single density-time curves. The latter reflects variation in contrast within a region of interest. As a result, washout curves from cardiac chambers for fractional volume measurements can be obtained.[55] In addition, DSA images using the radial shortening method have been satisfactorily used for analysis of segmental function. Functional or parametric images have been created to assess segmental contraction, amplitude of contraction, and synchrony or asynchrony of the contraction of the left ventricle.[19,51,52,54]

Cardiac catheterization in infants or small children is seldom indicated for the sole purpose of assessing left ventricular pump and contractile muscle function. Indeed, noninvasive methods, particularly echocardiography, are well suited for initial and serial determinations of simple indices of pump function such as shortening fraction, ejection fraction, and mean velocity of circumferential fiber shortening.[56–58] These noninvasive methods may also be applied to the estimation of contractile muscle function.[59]

However, sophisticated analyses of left ventricular pump and contractile function for clinical or research purposes may be desired during routinely scheduled catheterization. Evaluation of chamber size, ejection fraction, or mean velocity of circumferential fiber shortening requires adequate opacification of the left ventricular cavity over several cardiac cycles. The latter is necessary in order to obtain a representative number of biplane end-diastolic and end-systolic images for geometric volume determinations. Frame-by-frame evaluation of contractile function through analyses of wall stress and the end-systolic stress-volume relation further demands the integration of chamber volume and pressure data acquired at rapid frame rates in varying afterloaded states[60,61] (Fig. 8). This is a method that may require multiple injections of contrast medium. Despite these formidable obstacles, conventional left ventricular catheterization and angiography have provided a wealth of data in the adult patient.[62–65]

Similar efforts in children are rare and limited in scope.[66–68] Among the many concerns are: (1) the additional radiation exposure to the child which is needed to acquire the necessary biplane cine' images; (2) the volume of contrast medium needed for the analyses (adding to or subtracting from the amount of contrast agent intended for anatomic imaging); (3) the effects of repeated administration of contrast medium on left ventricular function[69,70]; and (4) the frequent occurrence of dysrhythmias following the injection of contrast medium directly into the left ventricle. These concerns are addressed by the DSA method, which minimizes or eliminates these problems and enables an experienced individual to plan and perform detailed studies of left ventricular pump and contractile function.

The method for performing these studies may be carried out in a variety of ways, but all share features common to the procedure we currently employ. We utilize a Philips (Philips Medical Systems, Inc., Shelton, CT) single-plane DSA system (DVI-2) equipped with an offline image processing system (APU).

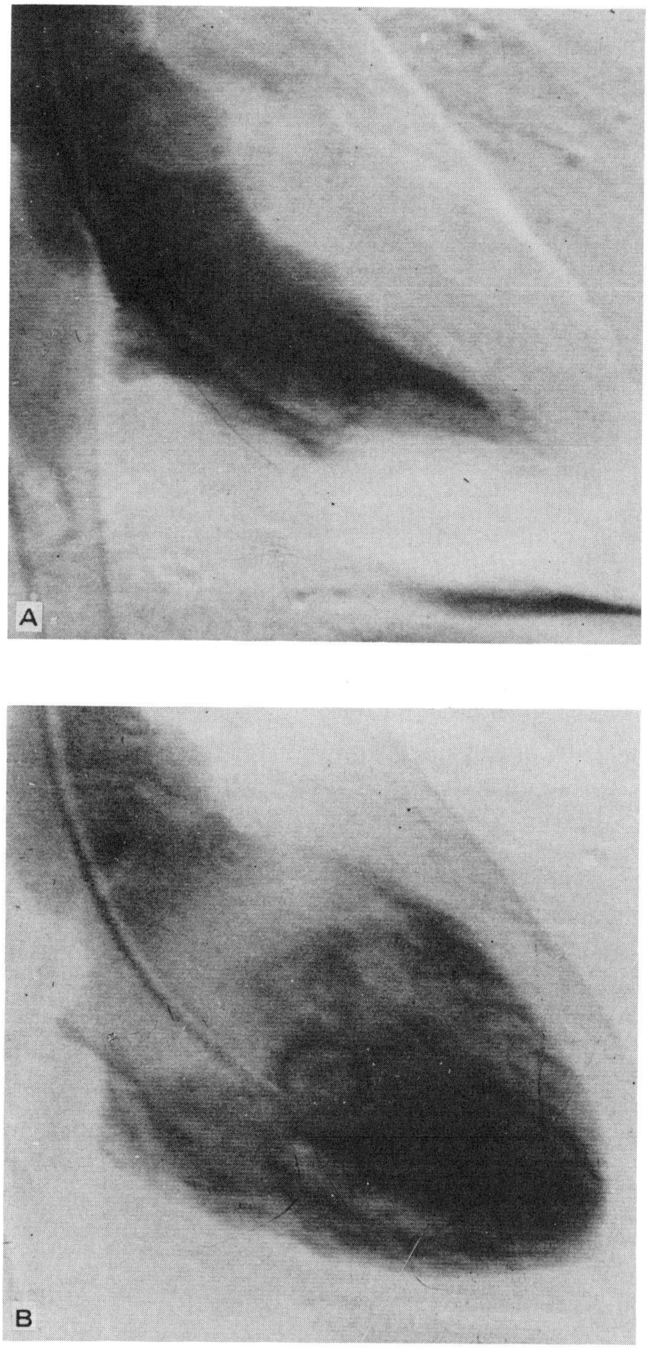

*FIGURE 8. A normal functional analysis. In this case, contrast medium was injected into the left ventricle via a 6 high-flow pigtail catheter. DSA images were obtained at end-systole (**A**) and at end-diastole (**B**). Planimetry of the left ventricle in each image was carried out manually and a composite image made (**C**). The ejection fraction was calculated by computer. After selecting the desired number of "compartments" to be analyzed, regional wall motion was calculated by the computer (**D**). Cardiac output can also be calculated by the computer if additional data, i.e., heart rate, are entered into the computer.*

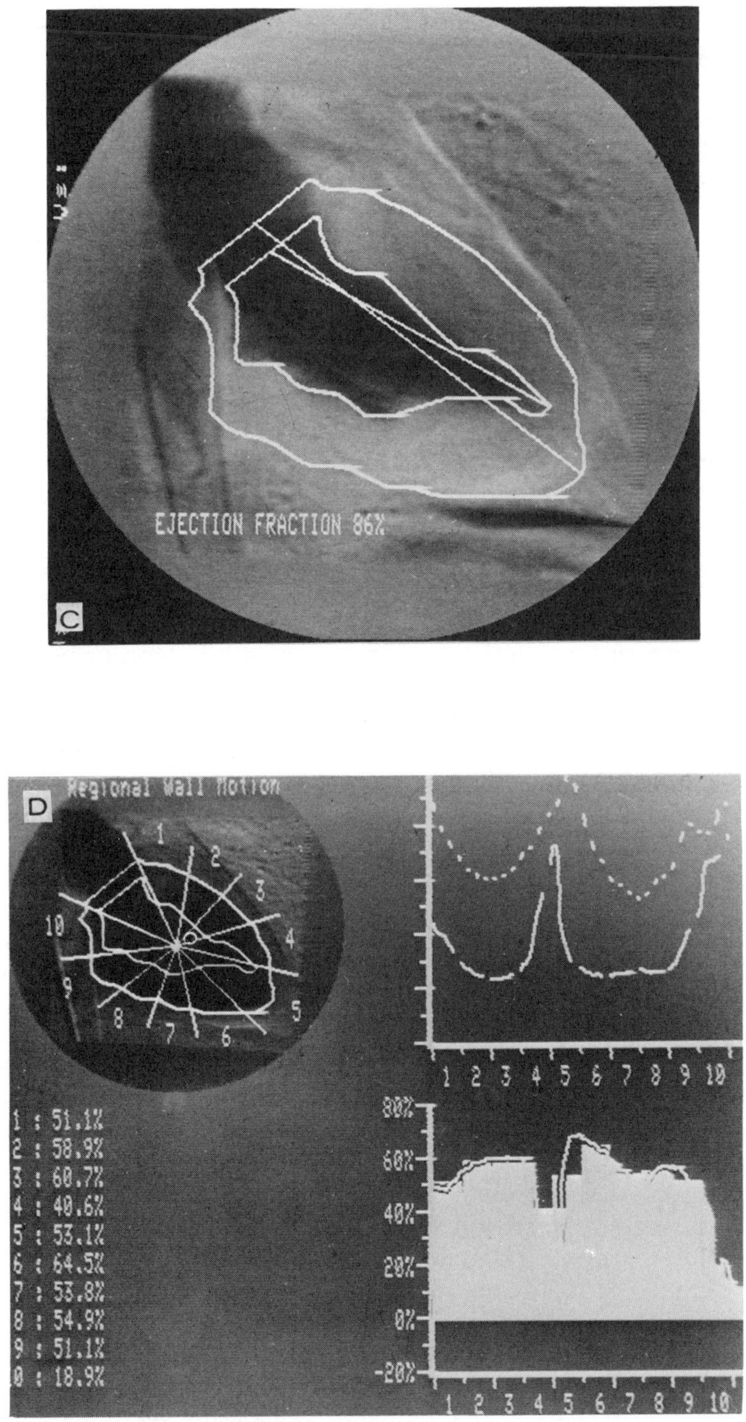
EJECTION FRACTION 86%
C
Regional Wall Motion
D
1 : 51.1%
2 : 58.9%
3 : 60.7%
4 : 40.6%
5 : 53.1%
6 : 64.5%
7 : 53.8%
8 : 54.9%
9 : 51.1%
0 : 18.9%
1 2 3 4 5 6 7 8 9 10
80%
60%
40%
20%
0%
-20%
1 2 3 4 5 6 7 8 9 10

Figures 8C, D.

A small amount of 70% Hypaque (0.2–0.5 mL/kg) is injected in the main pulmonary artery and the levophase is recorded on videotape in biplane fluoroscopy mode at the standard 30 video frames (60 video fields) per second. The images obtained by this method require a fraction of the usual cineradiation dose and extrasystoles seldom occur.

Simultaneous recording of the intraventricular pressure is made in analog format and indexed to the video frames by a timing signal that is added to the pressure recording and each video field in real time. This procedure is then repeated at varying afterloads created by inflating a large balloon in the descending aorta. Although studies are incomplete, there is some evidence that suggests that the small amounts of contrast medium used for these functional studies will have a negligible effect on the myocardium.[71]

Videotape processing on the offline system begins by converting the video analog signal to digital format using software which in our case is supplied by Philips Medical Systems, Inc. A 250 × 250 pixel matrix is constructed from each standard video frame by digitizing each video field and recombining the fields into a single digital frame (one digital frame is composed of two successive digital fields which are interlaced by alternating lines from each field). An appropriate mask is selected and subtraction is performed in the simple mask mode. Although a time-interval difference (TID) subtraction mode is occasionally used, we have not encountered significant problems with patient or respiratory motion. In addition, we have not found it necessary to perform pixel shifting or selective subtraction of different masks obtained over the respiratory cycle.[62]

Detailed study of contractile function requires analysis of pressure and volume data obtained at a minimum of 60 images/sec. In other methods, this has been achieved by converting single cineimages (recorded at 60 frames/sec) to a digital video format.[71] In our system, this requirement may be satisfied by simply separating each subtracted digital frame into its component digital fields. This reduces the resolution in the Y dimension (image top to bottom) by half; however, the large ventricular size and high pixel density make this a minor problem. Manual or automated planimetry of left ventricular borders is performed on corresponding anteroposterior and lateral digital fields, appropriate volume algorithms are applied, and indices of pump function are calculated[72,73] (Fig. 8). The latter have correlated well with standard left ventriculography, but differences in technique make direct comparison difficult.[74] Lastly, the volume and pressure data are recombined to yield parameters of contractile function. The entire process of digital subtraction, field separation, planimetry, volume calculation, and pressure-volume computations is accomplished expeditiously by menu-driven, user-designed software.

The ability to convert standard video analog images to digital format at 60 fields/sec permits virtually any video angiogram to be analyzed in the above manner. This is especially useful for research applications in animal studies where video images are obtained in a remote laboratory not equipped with DSA. In laboratories equipped with biplane DSA or for those applications requiring only single-plane analysis, digital images may be acquired directly without the need for video analog-to-digital conversion.

Advantages of Digital Subtraction Angiocardiography

By virtue of more sensitive detectors, computer conversion of transmitted x-rays to digital values and arithmetic manipulation of data, digital subtraction angiocardiography affords several distinct advantages over conventional angiocardiography[35, 36]:

1) significantly smaller amounts of contrast medium can be used as detection of low concentration of the contrast agent are enhanced and readily detected
2) overlying structures concealing opacified regions of interest can be removed by the subtraction technique improving visualization of pertinent anatomy and thus aid in arriving at an accurate diagnosis
3) the recorded study data can be manipulated to provide quality images for anatomic diagnosis as well as for functional analysis
4) the radiation dose can be reduced in comparison to conventional angiocardiography

Disadvantages of Digital Subtraction Angiocardiography

1) ionizing radiation produced
2) invasive procedure with some risks similar to those of conventional angiocardiography
3) equipment expensive
4) limitations of current equipment
   a) limited storage capacity may necessitate additional expensive disk storage alternatives
   b) archiving a major problem
      –magnetic tape cumbersome and impractical
      –videotape is an alternative but resolution decreased
5) voluntary or involuntary motion compromises image quality

Radiation Exposure

Whether angiocardiography is performed using conventional or digital subtraction techniques, the child will be exposed to ionizing radiation. The radiation dose using digital subtraction techniques can, at times, be less than that of conventional methods, although this will depend on a number of factors.

If IVDSA is utilized, the total radiation dose the child receives will be less than if conventional cineangiocardiography is performed. To put this into perspective, comparisons have been made between the radiation exposure from a chest radiograph with that from cardiac catheterization. The average dose absorbed by the chest of a child during a regular chest radiograph is 24 mR. In the case of cardiac catheterization, the chest absorbs an average of 5,810 mR during fluoroscopy and 1,592 mR during cineangiography. Therefore, the radiation dose[75] to the child's chest as a result of the fluoroscopy is equivalent to an average of 428.2 chest x-ray films and an average of 99.9 chest films as a result of the cineangiography. Obviously, the radiation dose is significantly increased when using biplane fluoroscopy and cineangiography.[76]

The radiation dose measured by the incident surface exposure during IVDSA approximates that of conventional cineangiography.[77] The amount of fluoroscopy time utilized during IVDSA, however, is considerably less than that used during conventional intra-arterial studies when more fluoroscopy time is used during the passing, manipulation, and relocation of catheters in the vessels or cardiac chambers.

As has been noted previously, IVDSA is not the method of choice in the evaluation of congenital heart disease and particularly not for cases of complex congenital heart defects. In most instances, DSA will be substituted for cineangiocardiography during the cardiac catheterization procedure. Therefore, the radiation dose received by the patient during the catheterization procedure will be unchanged. If digital subtraction imaging is used in place of cineimaging the radiation dose may be reduced. The three most commonly used methods to reduce the radiation exposure to the patient are pulsed imaging, temporal averaging, and recursive filtering.[78] Much of this depends on the type of equipment used. A practical procedure that the angiographer can follow in order to decrease the radiation exposure to the patient is to use the lowest frame rate possible to achieve a diagnostic study.

References

1. Kelley MJ, Jaffee CC, Kleinman CS: *Cardiac Imaging in Infants and Children*. Philadelphia, PA: W.B. Saunders Co. 1982, pp. 1–3.
2. Arey JB: *Cardiovascular Pathology in Infants and Children*. Philadelphia, PA: W.B. Saunders Co. 1984, pp. 31–54.
3. MacMahon B, McKeown T, Record RG: The incidence and life expectation of children with congenital heart disease. *Br Heart J* 15:121–129, 1954.
4. Grigg ERN: *The Trail of the Invisible Light*. Springfield, MA: Charles C. Thomas Publisher. 1965, pp. 616–618.
5. Capp MP, Ovitt TW: Digital angiography in the diagnosis of congenital heart disease: An alternative viewpoint. *Cardiovasc Interven Radiol* 7:190–191, 1984.
6. Higgins CB, Berger H, Boyd D, et al: Cardiovascular radiology. *Invest Radiol* 19:1–7, 1984.
7. Wholey MH: Cardiovascular applications of digital subtraction angiography. *Radiol Clin North Am* 23:627–639, 1985.
8. Barron JV, Sahn DJ, Valdes-Cruz LM, et al: Clinical utility of two-dimensional Doppler echocardiographic techniques for estimating pulmonary to systemic flow ratio in children with left to right shunting, atrial septal defect, ventricular septal defect, and patent ductus arteriosus. *J Am Coll Cardiol* 3:169–175, 1984.
9. Lipton MJ: Quantitation of cardiac function by Cine'-CT. *Radiol Clin North Am* 23:613–626, 1985.
10. Soulen RL, Donner RMM: Magnetic resonance imaging of rerouted pulmonary blood flow. *Radiol Clin North Am* 23:737–744, 1985.

11. Miller W, Brady RJ, Dinsmore RE, et al: Cardiac magnetic resonance imaging: The Massachusetts General Hospital experience. *Radiol Clin North Am* 23:745–746, 1985.
12. Heintzen PH, Brennecke R, Bursch JH: Improved safety by computerized video-angiocardiography. *Ann Radiol* 22:349–350, 1979.
13. Yiannikas J, Moodie DS, Gill CC: Pre and postoperative assessment of patients with left-to-right shunts using digital subtraction angiography (abstract). *Circulation* (Suppl), 66:II–104, 1982.
14. Moodie DS, Yiannikas J, Gill CC: Intravenous digital subtraction angiography in the evaluation of congenital abnormalities of the aorta and aortic arch. (abstract) *Circulation* (Suppl), 66:II–104, 1982.
15. Chung KJ, Hesselink JR, Chernoff HL: Digital subtraction angiography in patients with transposition of great arteries after surgical repair. (Abstract) *Circulation* (Suppl II) 66:11–104, 1982.
16. Brennecke R, Bursch JH, Bogren HG, et al: Digital intravenous imaging techniques in pediatric cardiology. In Mistretta CA, Crummy AB, Strother CM, Sachett JF (Eds): *Digital Subtraction Arteriography: An Application Of Computerized Fluoroscopy*. Chicago, IL: Year Book Medical Publishers, 1982, pp. 133–141.
17. Reiderer SJ: Digital radiography. In Taveras JM, Ferrucci JT (Eds): *Radiology, Diagnosis-Imaging-Intervention* vol. 1. Philadelphia, PA, J.B. Lippincott Co.: 1985, pp. 1–11.
18. Kyung JC, Hesselink JR: Review of digital subtraction angiography in the diagnosis of congenital heart disease. *Cardiovasc Interven Radiol* 7:188–189, 1984.
19. Higgins CB, Buonocore E: Digital subtraction angiography. In Friedman WF, Higgins CB (Eds): *Pediatric Cardiac Imaging*. Philadelphia, PA: W.B. Saunders Co., 1984, pp. 51–63.
20. Fletcher BD, Jacobstein MD, Morrison SC: Intravenous digital subtraction angiography (IVDSA) in children. *Pediatr Radiol* 14:425–430, 1984.
21. Capitanio MA, Faerber EN, Gainey MA, et al: Digital subtraction angiography and its application in children. *Pediatr Clin North Am* 32:1449–1459, 1985.
22. Amundson GM, Wesenberg RL, Mueller DL, et al: Pediatric digital subtraction angiography. *Radiology* 153:649–654, 1984.
23. Grossman LB, Buonocore D, Modic MT, et al: Digital subtraction angiography of the thoracic aorta. *Radiology* 150:323–325, 1984.
24. Moodie DS, Yiannikas J, Gill CC, et al: Intravenous digital subtraction angiography in the evaluation of congenital abnormalities of the aorta and aortic arch. *Am Heart J* 104:628–634, 1982.
25. Mancini GBJ, Ostrander DR, Slutsky RA, et al: Intravenous versus left ventricular injection of ionic contrast material: Hemodynamic implications for digital subtraction angiography. *AJR* 140:425–430, 1983.
26. Panuel M, Devred P, Girard N, et al: Digitalized angiography of the thorax in children. *J Radiol* 67:25–30, 1986.
27. Tonkin ILD, Gold RE, Moser D, et al: Evaluation of vascular rings with digital subtraction angiography. *AJR* 142:1287–1291, 1984.
28. Kruger RA, Anderson RE, Koehler PR, et al: Methods for the noninvasive evaluation of cardiovascular dynamics using a digital radiographic device. *Radiology* 139:301–305, 1981.
29. Hardin CW, Kruger RA, Anderson FL, et al: Real-time digital angiography using a temporal high-pass filter. *Radiology* 151:517–520, 1984.
30. Crummy AB, Strother CM, Sackett JF, et al: Computerized fluoroscopy: Digital subtraction for intravenous angiocardiography and arteriography. *AJR* 135:1131–1140, 1980.
31. Bogren HG, Seibert JA, Hines HH, et al: The beneficial effects of short pulse width acquisition and ECG-gating in digital angiocardiography. *Invest Radiol* 19:284–290, 1984.
32. Mistretta CA, Andrew B: Diagnosis of cardiovascular disease by digital subtraction angiography. *Science* 214:761–765, 1981.

33. Kruger RA, Mistretta A, Houk TL, et al: Computerized fluoroscopy in real-time noninvasive visualization of the cardiovascular system. *Radiology* 130:49–57, 1979.
34. Brennecke R, Brown TK, Bursch J, et al: Computerized video image processing with application to cardioangiographic roentgen image series. In Hagel HH (Ed): *Digital Image Processing*. New York: Springer-Verlag, 1977, p. 244.
35. Bursch JH: Digital angiocardiography for assessment of congenital heart disease. In Friedman WF, Higgins CB (Eds): *Pediatric Cardiac Imaging*. Philadelphia, PA: W.B. Saunders Co., 1984, pp. 64–75.
36. Buonocore E, Pavlicek WA, Modic MT, et al: Anatomic and functional imaging of congenital heart disease with digital subtraction angiography. *Radiology* 147:647–654, 1983.
37. Bogren HG, Bursch JH: Digital angiography in the diagnosis of congenital heart disease. *Cardiovasc Interven Radiol* 7:180–188, 1984.
38. Dickinson DF, Wilson N, Partridge JB: Digital subtraction angiography in infants and children with congenital heart disease. *Br Heart J* 51:485–491, 1984.
39. Tonkin IL: Digital subtraction angiography in congenital heart disease. *Semin Roentgenol* 20:283–289, 1985.
40. Partridge JB, Dickinson DF: Digital subtraction angiography (DSA) in congenital heart disease. *Electromedia* 51:148–151, 1983.
41. Levin AR, Goldberg HL, Borer JS, et al: Digital angiography in the pediatric patient with congenital heart disease: Comparison with standard methods. *Circulation* 68:374–384, 1983.
42. Moodie DS: Assessing cardiac anatomy with digital subtraction angiography. *J Am Coll Cardiol* 5:485–545, 1985.
43. Tobis JM, Henry WL, Nalcioglu O: Cardiac applications of digital subtraction angiography. *Appl Radiol/Cardiac Imaging* 61–67, 1983.
44. Tonkin IL, Fitch SJ, Magill HL, et al: Pediatric digital subtraction angiography: Intraarterial and intracardiac applications. *Pediatr Radiol* 16:126–130, 1986.
45. Bargeron LM Jr, Elliot LP, Soto B, et al: Axial angiography in congenital heart disease. I. Concept, technical and anatomic considerations. *Circulation* 56:1075–1093, 1977.
46. Vogel M, Sebening W, Schumacher G, et al: Clinical uses of digital subtraction angiography for imaging anatomy immediately following heart operations in childhood. *Herz* 10:201–207, 1985.
47. Yiannikas J, Moodie DS, Dill CC, et al: Intravenous digital subtraction angiography in the assessment of patients with left to right shunts before and after surgical correction. *J Am Coll Cardiol* 3:1507–1514, 1984.
48. Yiannikas J, Moodie DS, Sterba R, et al: Intravenous digital subtraction angiography to assess pre- and postoperatively aneurysms of the ventricular and atrial septum. *Am J Cardiol* 53:383–385, 1984.
49. Buonocore E: Digital subtraction angiography of the heart. RSNA Radiologic Study Programs RSP 260, 1986.
50. Maltz DL, Treves S: Quantitative radionuclide angiocardiography: Determination of Qp:Qs in children. *Circulation* 47:1049–1054, 1973.
51. Bursch JH, Heintzen PH: Parametric Imaging. *Radiol Clin North Am* 23:321–333, 1985.
52. Higgins CB, Norris SL, Gerber KH, et al: Quantitation of the left ventricular dimensions and function by digital video subtraction angiography. *Radiology* 144:461–469, 1982.
53. Kruger RA, Anderson RE, Koehler PR, et al: A method for the noninvasive evaluation of cardiovascular dynamics using a digital radiographic device. *Radiology* 139:301–305, 1981.
54. Newell JD, Kelley MJ, Ovitt TW: Digital cardiac radiology. *Radiol Clin North Am* 23:261–273, 1985.
55. Lange PE, Budach W, Radtke W, et al: Right ventricular imaging with digital subtraction angiocardiography using intraventricular contrast injection. *Am J Cardiol* 54:839–842, 1984.

56. Sahn DJ, Deely WJ, Hagan AD, et al: Echocardiographic assessment of left ventricular performance in normal newborns. *Circulation* 49:232–236, 1974.
57. Meyer RA, Stockert J, Kaplan S: Echographic determination of left ventricular volumes in pediatric patients. *Circulation* 51:297–303, 1975.
58. Disessa TG, Kirkman JH, Ching CT, et al: Evaluation of cardiac chamber size and left ventricular function in children using two-dimensional apex echocardiography. *Am J Cardiol* 45:468, 1980.
59. Borow KM, Green LH, Grossman W: Left ventricular end-systolic stress-shortening and stress-length relations in humans. *Am J Cardiol* 50:1301–1308, 1982.
60. Hood, WP, Rackley CE, Rolett ET: Wall stress in the normal and hypertrophied human left ventricle. *Am J Cardiol* 22:550–558, 1968.
61. Mehmel HC, Stockins B, Ruffmann K, et al: The linearity of the end-systolic pressure-volume relationship in man and its sensitivity for assessment of left ventricular function. *Circulation* 63:1216–1222, 1981.
62. Carabello BA, Green LH, Grossman W, et al: Hemodynamic determinants of prognosis of aortic valve replacement in critical aortic stenosis and advanced congestive heart failure. *Circulation* 62:42–48, 1980.
63. Huber D, Grimm J, Koch R, et al: Determinants of ejection performance in aortic stenosis. *Circulation* 64:126–134, 1981.
64. Carabello BA, Nolan SP, McGuire LB: Assessment of preoperative left ventricular function in patients with mitral regurgitation: Value of the end-systolic wall stress-end-systolic volume ratio. *Circulation* 64:1212–1217, 1981.
65. Carabello BA, Gash A, Mayer D, et al: Normal left ventricular systolic function in adults with atrial septal defect and left heart failure. *Am J Cardiol* 49:1868–1873, 1982.
66. Jarmakani MM, Edwards SB, Spach MS, et al: Left ventricular pressure-volume characteristics in congenital heart disease. *Circulation* 37:879–889, 1968.
67. Donner RM, Carabello BA, Black IN, et al: Left ventricular wall stress in compensated aortic stenosis in children. *Am J Cardiol* 51:946–951, 1982.
68. Donner RM, Black In, Spann JF, et al: Left ventricular wall stress and function in childhood coarctation of the aorta. *J Am Coll Cardiol* 5:1161–1167, 1985.
69. Brown R, Rahimtoola SH, Davis GD, et al: The effect of angiocardiographic contrast medium on circulatory dynamics in man. *Circulation* 31:234–240, 1965.
70. Freisinger GC, Schaffer J, Criley JM, et al: Hemodynamic consequences of the injection of radiopaque material. *Circulation* 31:730–740, 1965.
71. Sasayama S, Nonogi H, Kawai C, et al: Automated method for left ventricular volume measurement by cineventriculography with minimal doses of contrast medium. *Am J Cardiol* 48:746–753, 1981.
72. Heintzen PH, Bursch HJ, Hahne HJ, et al: Assessment of cardiovascular function by digital angiography. *J Am Coll Cardiol* 5:150S–157S, 1985.
73. Graham TP, Jarmakani JM, Canent RV, et al: Left heart volume estimation in infancy and childhood. *Circulation* 43:895–904, 1971.
74. Norris SL, Slutsky RA, Mancini GBJ, et al: Comparison of digital intravenous ventriculography with direct left ventriculography for quantitation of left ventricular volumes and ejection fractions. *Am J Cardiol* 51:1399–1403, 1983.
75. Walman JD, Rummerfield PS, Gilpin EA, et al: Radiation exposure to the child during cardiac catheterization. *Circulation* 64:158–163, 1981.
76. Leibovic SJ, Fellows KE: Patient radiation exposure during cardiac catheterization. *Cardiovasc Interven Radiol* 6:150–153, 1983.
77. Fletcher BD: Digital x-ray imaging techniques in pediatric diagnosis. *Am J Dis Child* 136:771–773, 1982.
78. Rimkus K, Baily NA: Patient exposure requirements for high contrast resolution in digital radiographic systems. *AJR* 142:603–608, 1984.

Chapter 5

Digital Subtraction Angiography of the Aorta and Great Vessels

INA L.D. TONKIN

Digital subtraction angiography (DSA) is now a routine vascular imaging modality for adults, and is gaining increased acceptance in diagnostic and therapeutic angiographic applications in children.[1–7] Reports indicate diagnostic images with intravenous DSA in the evaluation of congenital anomalies of the aorta and in aortic dissection in adults.[8–11] In addition, intra-arterial digital subtraction angiography is diagnostic for anomalies of the thoracic aorta in children.[6] Digital imaging has become a complementary technique for cardiac catheterization in children and is particularly helpful in interventional radiologic procedures.[12–14]

Digital subtraction angiography is utilized in all vascular procedures at LeBonheur Children's Medical Center and patients evaluated from St. Jude Children's Research Hospital. In addition, approximately one third of all patients evaluated for diagnostic or interventional procedures in congenital heart disease are imaged with DSA techniques. DSA is now utilized routinely in many centers for the diagnostic evaluation of cardiac disease.[15–19]

DSA Systems

During the past five years, we have evaluated all pediatric patients undergoing vascular and/or interventional procedures with digital subtraction angiography. In many children's medical centers, the hospital may maximize their facilities by conducting both angiographic and interventional procedures in a single room along with a cardiac catheterization laboratory. Our dual-room facility allows digital imaging in both a special procedures and interventional laboratory as well as in a dedicated cardiac catheterization laboratory, which alleviates scheduling difficulties.

Digital Subtraction Imaging in Infants and Children, edited by Eric N. Faerber. Mount Kisco, New York: Futura Publishing Company, Inc., © 1989.

Basic to any angiographic room is a high-quality fluoroscopic system, a programmable film changer, a three-phased generator, x-ray tube with a high heat rating and variable focal spot size, and power contrast material injectors. The pediatric patient can be evaluated with a 6.5- or 9.0-inch image intensifier and the entire thoracic or abdominal aorta can be imaged in most patients. The 14-inch image intensifier required for abdominal and extremity vascular imaging in the adult is not necessary for most pediatric patients. All rooms should be equipped with ECG monitors and the supplies necessary for advanced life support.

The image intensifier should be mounted on an arm capable of complex angulation. A parallelogram, C-arm, or L/U configuration is extremely useful, especially if mounted on an arm that moves rapidly and easily around the patient. This obviates the need to move seriously ill patients or uncooperative small children. It also enables rapid and more precise visualization of overlapping vessels. C-arms or parallelograms are essential in evaluating complex congenital heart lesions because they allow the C-arm to be placed perpendicular to the cardiac axis for optimal imaging.[19]

In the cardiac catheterization laboratory, Philips Poly Diagnost C (Philips Medical Systems, Inc., Shelton, CT) radiographic imaging equipment is utilized with biplane cinefilming at 30, 60, or 90 frames per second (fps). The ADAC Digital Radiography Processing System 4100 Camera (ADAC Laboratories, San Jose, CA) is mounted on the image intensifier (6.5- and 9-inch) so that only single-plane DSA is currently available in the cardiac catheterization laboratory imaging at 30 images/second with a 256 × 256 × 8 bit matrix.

In the special procedures room, a Philips UPI C-arm is utilized with a three film/second puck changer. In this laboratory, DSA images can be obtained with the 512 × 512 × 8 bit matrix at a rate of 5 images/sec. We hope to upgrade one or both laboratories within the near future. A remote acquisition terminal is stationed between the two laboratories for acquisition of images.

In all patients, a 3–5 F Cook (Cook, Inc., Bloomington, IN) or Mallinckrodt (Mallinckrodt, Inc., St. Louis, MO) high-flow catheter was used. Patients were sedated with an intramuscular injection of Demerol (1–2 mg/kg), Phenergan (0.5 mg/kg), and Thorazine (0.5 mg/kg). Bolus injections ranged from 0.5 to 1.0 cc/kg of diatrizoate meglumine 76 for each injection, with dilution of contrast material by 50% or 75% with heparinized bacteriostatic water. During the last 3½ years, Hexabrix (ioxaglate meglumine 39.3% and ioxaglate sodium 19.6%), a low osmolality contrast agent was used 50% diluted with heparinized bacteriostatic water.[20–21] The use of low osmolality contrast material has decreased misregistration of the digital images and motion artifacts.

During the last four years, approximately one third of patients evaluated with DSA have been studied with a day care admission and are discharged at the end of the day with arterial or venous catheterizations. Patients may be studied in an outpatient setting because excellent digital images can be obtained using very small catheters and low volumes of contrast material. There have been no significant complications at our institution. The quality of the study is less dependent on patient cooperation with intra-arterial examinations using dilute, low osmolality, nonionic contrast material.[20] Therefore, the images are diagnostic in 90%–95% of all pediatric patients.

Aortic Arch Anomalies

While evaluating the types of equipment necessary for digital vascular imaging of the pediatric patient, we published our first series of seven patients with vascular rings using intravenous digital subtraction techniques. The systems used included CGR (Thompson, S. A., Paris, France, a division of GE, Milwaukee, WI), Diasonics (OEC-Diasonics, Inc., Salt Lake City, UT) and Philips DVI-I imaging systems.[10] Aortic arch anomalies can easily be evaluated with IV-DSA or IA-DSA (Fig. 1).

A Left Aortic Arch with an Aberrant Right Subclavian Artery

The anatomy is well demonstrated in this patient with a left aortic arch and an aberrant right subclavian artery. This aortic arch anomaly occurs in 1 in 200 individuals. This lesion is very, very rarely associated with a vascular ring or symptomatology. This aortic arch anomaly can be seen in patients with tetralogy of Fallot and coarctation of the aorta, as well as with ventricular septal defects (Fig. 1).

Double Aortic Arch

If a double aortic arch persists, a complete vascular ring occurs. Each arch passes over the homolateral bronchus, giving rise to a subclavian artery and a common carotid artery. All recorded cases to date have a left ductus arteriosus. The luminal size of the two arches varies; they may be equal in size but more frequently (80% of the cases) the right arch is larger than the left (Fig. 2). The left arch may be atretic.

Double aortic arch is the most common aortic arch anomaly to produce symptoms and require surgical correction. The infant may have stridor and dysphasia or recurrent aspiration pneumonia. Digital subtraction angiography is diagnostic in detecting aortic arch anomalies. Angled angiography can be performed to demonstrate the anatomy.[10]

Right Aortic Arch

The right-sided aortic arch is a fairly common aortic arch malformation occurring in 1 out of 2,500 persons. A right-sided aortic arch develops because of a break in the hypothetical double aortic arch. The type I aortic arch with mirror-image branching has a high association (approximately 85–90%) with congenital heart lesions such as tetralogy of Fallot, persistent truncus arteriosus, and tricuspid atresia. However, the most common type of right aortic arch visualized in the adult is the type II right aortic arch which has an aberrant left subclavian artery.

The right aortic arch with an aberrant left subclavian artery, short left ligamentum arteriosum, and right descending aorta may form a tight vascular ring or vascular compression anomaly around the esophagus and trachea in infancy causing stridor and dysphasia (Figs. 3–5). An esophagogram will show the right-sided indentation from the right aortic arch on the posterior-anterior projection with a posterior indentation on the barium-filled esophagus on the lateral view from the aberrant right subclavian artery and large aortic diverticulum (Fig. 3). The adult patient with this anomaly is asymptomatic, but a mediastinal mass may be suspected on the patient's plain chest radiograph. IA- or IV-DSA will demonstrate the classic right aortic arch with an aberrant left subclavian artery and aortic diverticulum. In this anomaly, the first branch is the left common carotid followed by the right common carotid artery, the right subclavian artery, and the fourth branch is the aberrant left subclavian artery. However, with symptoms of decreased radial artery pulse in the left arm, the classic web or stenosis of the aberrant left subclavian artery will be noted as it arises from the aortic diverticulum. This lesion is amenable to angioplasty or balloon dilatation procedure (Fig. 5).

An unusual vascular ring consisting of a right aortic arch with a diverticulum and ligamentum is also illustrated (Fig. 6).

Coarctation of the Aorta

Patients with coarctation of the aorta can easily be imaged with digital subtraction angiography (Fig. 7). Coarctation of the aorta is a congenital anomaly consisting of a focal narrowing of the aorta. In general, two types of coarctation are recognized: diffuse (preductal coarctation) and localized or discrete (juxtaductal or postductal type coarctation of the aorta). The discrete type is the most common form and consists of a localized infolding toward the lumen of all portions of the aorta (Fig. 7).[6]

Palliative Shunts in Congenital Heart Disease

In evaluating patients with congenital heart disease, DSA is used to determine the patency of vascular shunts such as a modified Blalock-Taussig anastomosis, a central shunt, and the Glenn procedure (Figs. 8, 9, and 10). This imaging technique is excellent for the visualization of extremely small left-to-right shunts such as in patients with coronary artery fistulas (Fig. 11). The resolution is 1.8–2.0 line pairs/mm with the 6.5-image intensifier and the 512 × 512 matrix.

Interrupted Aortic Arch

Complex aortic arch anomalies can be imaged with digital subtraction angiography and currently the cardiac catheterization laboratory can image patients at 30 images/sec with the 256 × 256 matrix. A patient with a complex interrupted aortic arch and truncus arteriosus was diagnosed with DSA (Fig. 12). In addition, another complex aortic arch anomaly consisting of an aorticopulmonary window with severe tetralogy of Fallot and pulmonary atresia was imaged with an aortic injection using digital subtraction angiography (Fig. 13).

Pulmonary Sequestration

Digital subtraction angiography has been an excellent imaging modality to evaluate patients with pulmonary sequestration (Fig. 14). The supplying artery is well imaged and the venous anatomy is even better demonstrated with contrast enhancement using digital subtraction angiographic techniques (Fig. 15).

Embolization Procedures

Digital angiography is also helpful in diagnosing sites of extravasation of contrast material secondary to hemorrhage in patients with hemoptysis. Bronchial artery embolization and aortography can be performed in patients with hemoptysis secondary to cystic fibrosis, chronic infection (tuberculosis, aspergillosis), or secondary to radiation therapy (Fig. 16). Extravasation can be visualized and embolization procedures can be controlled with this technique.

During embolization of hemorrhagic vessels, digital angiography allows rapid assessment of the extent of embolization. It will indicate when a satisfactory result has been achieved and avoid the complication of reflux embolization. Reflux emboli can occur with too vigorous an injection in an area of ongoing thrombolysis. In addition, the painless nature of digital imaging is valuable in those patients who must undergo serial vascular imaging. The total contrast volume is greatly decreased which further increases patient safety.

Conclusion

DSA is a safe diagnostic procedure in the pediatric age group. All children requiring angiographic evaluations of congenital anomalies of the aorta may be imaged with DSA techniques. These studies are now diagnostic. New technical developments will increase the advantages and applications of DSA for the pediatric patient.

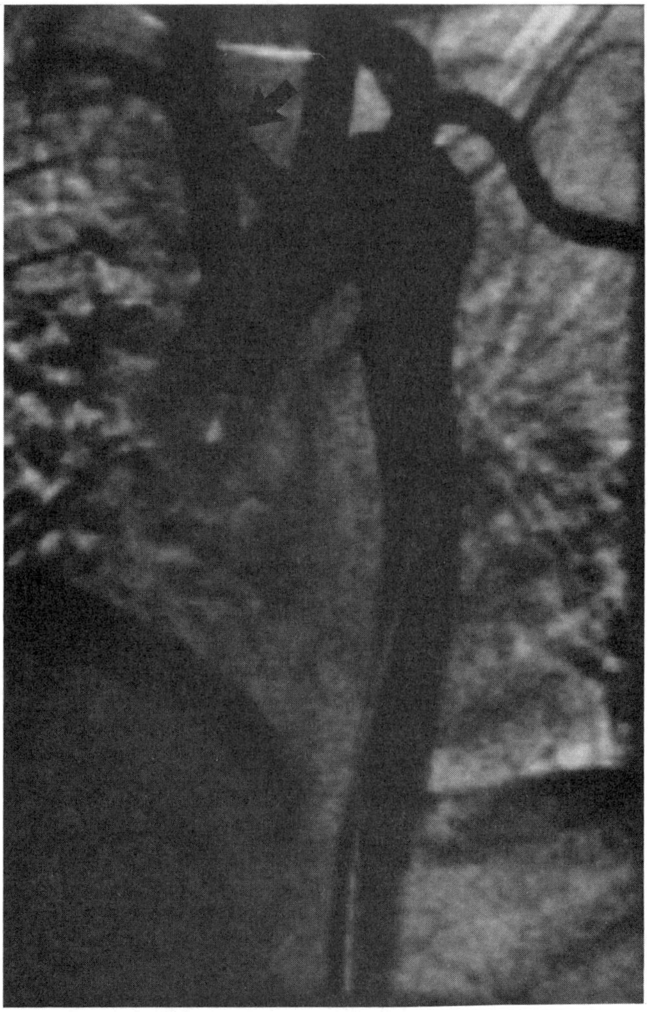

FIGURE 1. Aortogram in a 14-year-old white male with a perimembranous ventricular septal defect showed a left aortic arch with an aberrant right subclavian artery (arrow) imaged by IADSA. The catheter was placed in the ascending aorta. The LAO projection with cranial angulation was performed to unwind the left aortic arch. The first branch is the right common carotid artery, followed by the left common carotid artery, the left subclavian artery, and the last branch is the aberrant right subclavian artery.

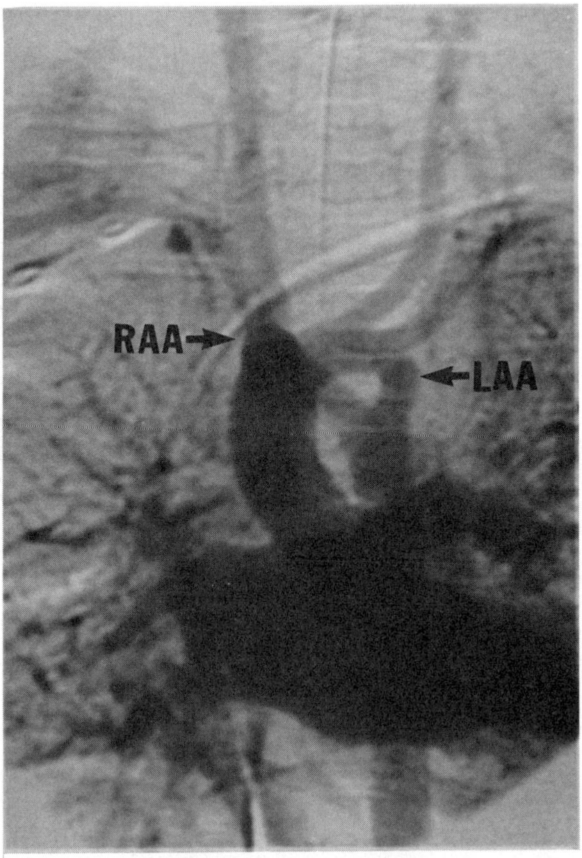

FIGURE 2. *Imaging of vascular rings or aortic arch anomalies. A two-month-old female with severe respiratory distress and hyperextension of the neck required intratracheal intubation. An esophagogram was compatible with a vascular ring. The IVDSA image with an injection into the right atrium showed an excellent example of the vascular anatomy. Note the double aortic arch with a high posterior right arch component (RAA, arrow) and a smaller but patent anterior left aortic arch component (arrow, LAA). This patient underwent a left thoracotomy for successful ligation of a double aortic arch. In addition, this patient underwent tracheal resection for severe tracheomalacia.*

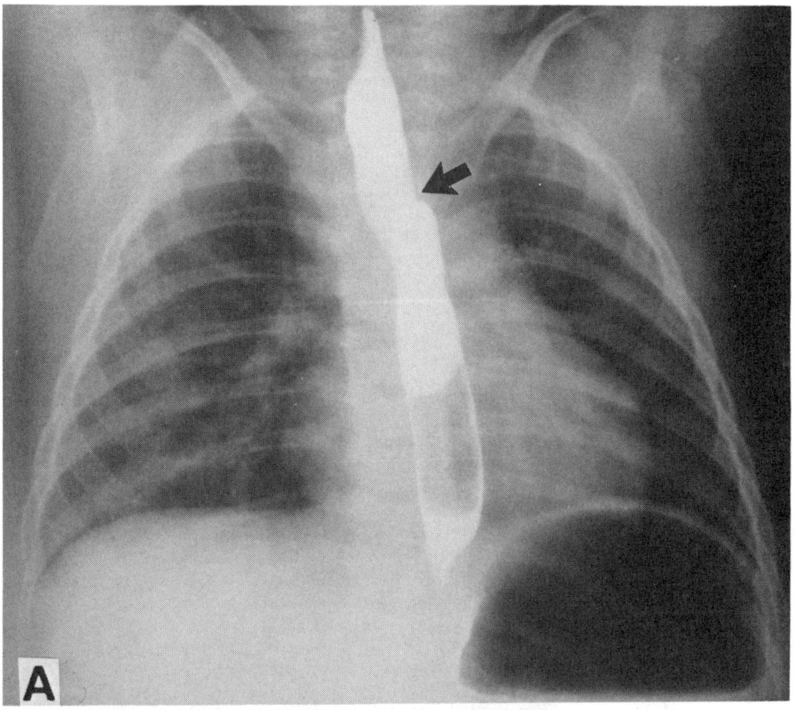

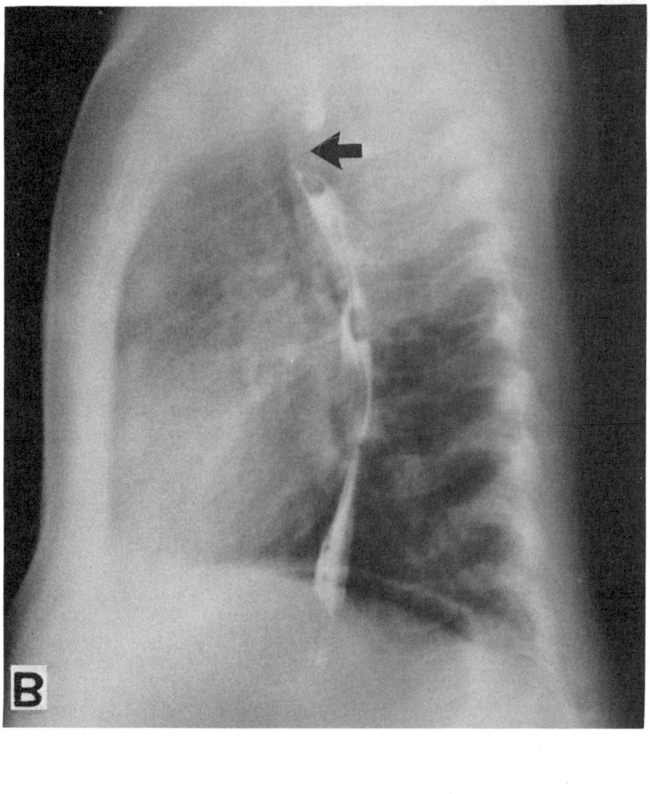

Figure 3A,B. ***A:*** *A five-month-old female presented with feeding difficulties in infancy. The PA esophagogram showed a right sided aortic arch with impressions on the barium filled esophagus (arrow).* ***B:*** *The lateral projection showed a posterior impression (arrow) on the barium-filled esophagus compatible with a vascular ring.*

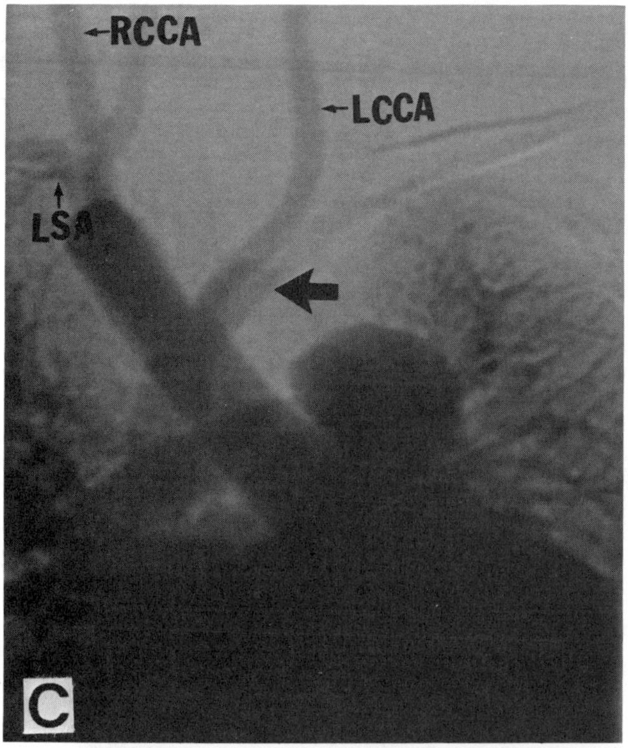

FIGURE 3C,D. *C: Intravenous digital subtraction angiography demonstrated the anatomy of the vascular ring. The patient has a right aortic arch with the first branch being the left common carotid artery (LCCA), followed by the right common carotid artery (RCCA), followed by the left subclavian artery (LSA). The last branch is the aberrant right subclavian artery (arrow). D: The long-axial, oblique projection of this same patient demonstrated the last branch to be the aberrant left subclavian artery (ALSA). In correlation with the esophagogram, the patient has a short ligamentum from the aberrant left subclavian artery to the left pulmonary artery to complete the vascular ring. The patient underwent a left thoracotomy for successful ligation of the vascular ring.*

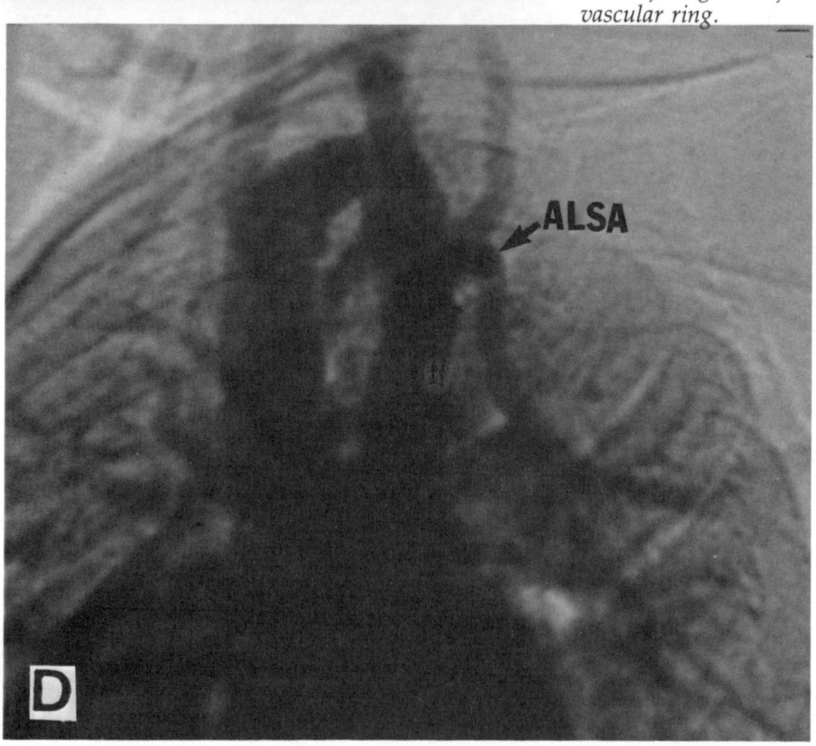

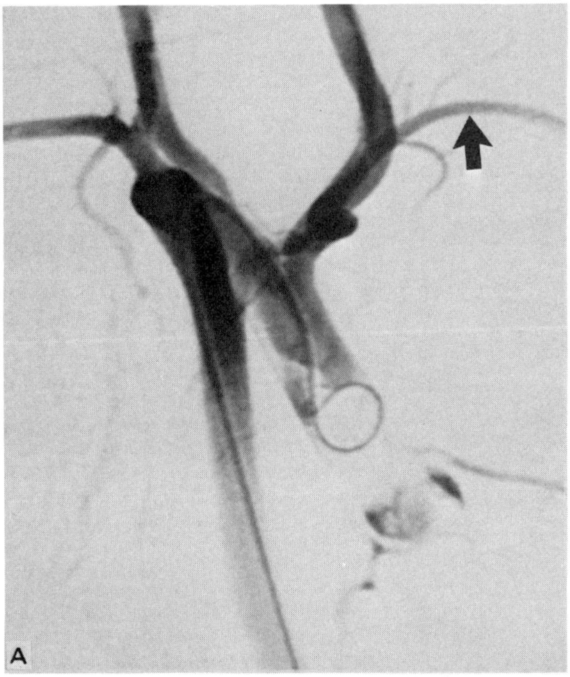

FIGURE 4A. A 10-month-old male with a history of hyaline membrane disease and bronchopulmonary dysplasia showed signs of continued respiratory distress with a right-sided aortic arch noted on the chest radiograph. An esophagogram showed a probable aberrant left subclavian artery or vascular ring. IADSA demonstrated the anatomy, showing a high right-sided aortic arch with an aberrant left subclavian artery (arrow).

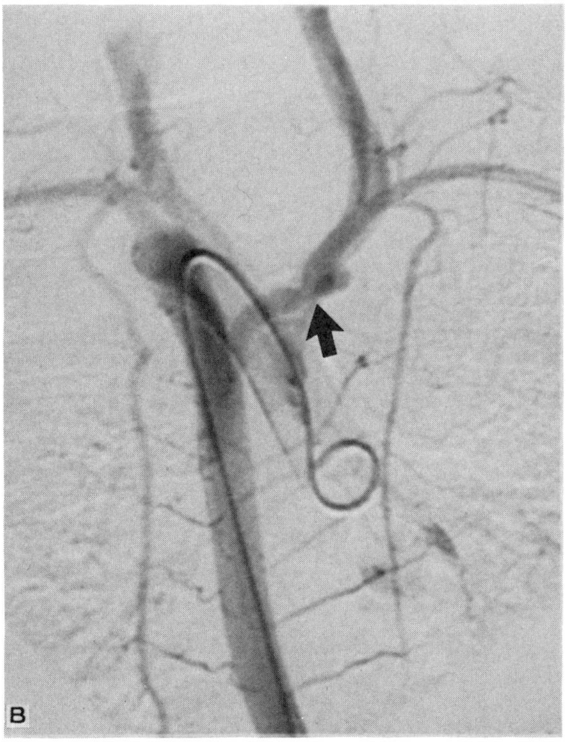

FIGURE 4B. An image obtained later in sequence demonstrated the aberrant left subclavian artery with a web or kink approximately 1 cm from its origin (arrow). At surgery, this was the ligamentous attachment from the aberrant left subclavian artery to the left pulmonary artery completing the vascular ring.

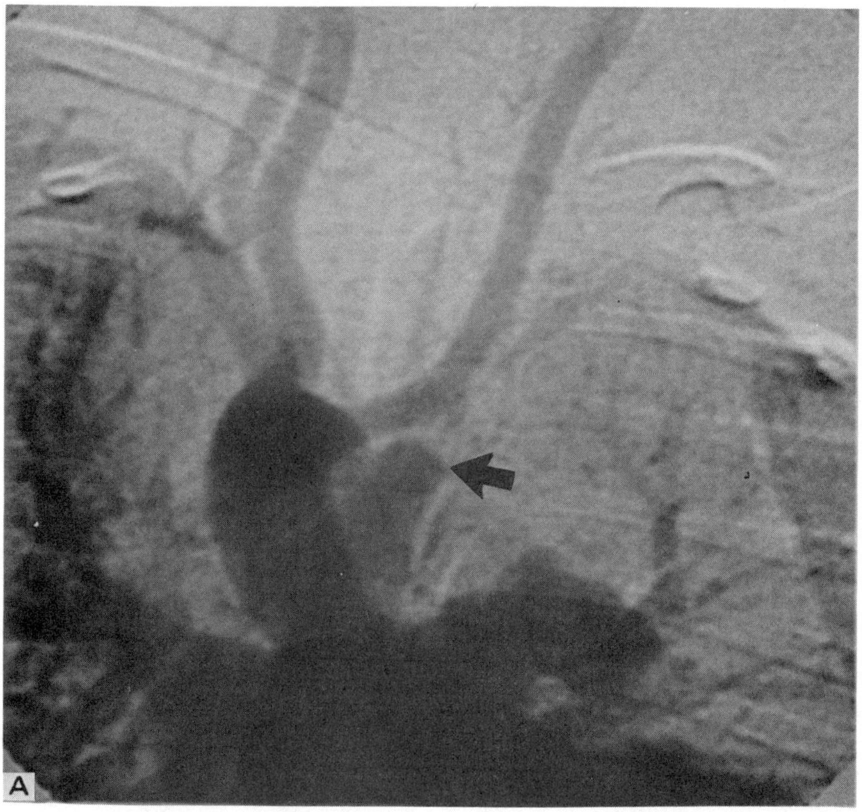

FIGURE 5A. *The intravenous DSA of a five-month-old male who presented with stridor, showed a large right-sided aortic arch with a left diverticulum (arrow). The esophagogram was compatible with a form of vascular ring.*

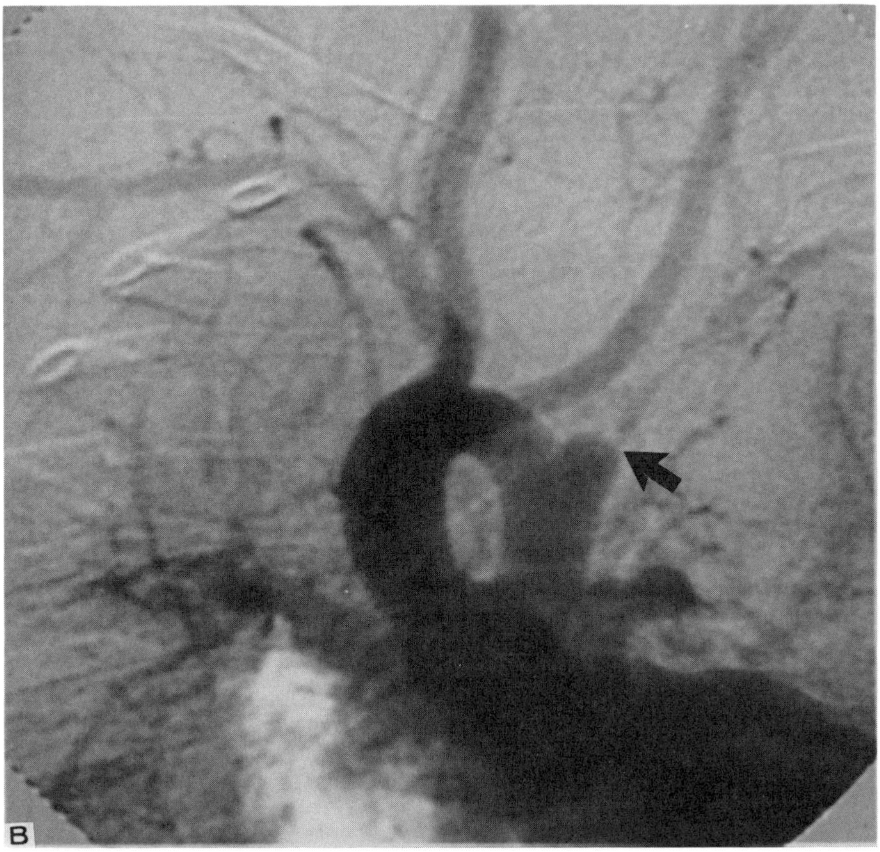

FIGURE 5B. The left anterior oblique projection demonstrated a right aortic arch with an aberrant left subclavian artery (arrow). Note the aberrant left subclavian artery is hypoplastic rising from the aortic diverticulum. There are also aortic collaterals to this left subclavian artery. There is a short ligamentum from the aberrant subclavian to the left pulmonary artery which completes the vascular ring. This patient underwent surgical correction of the vascular ring with a left thoracotomy approach. There was an excellent surgical result.

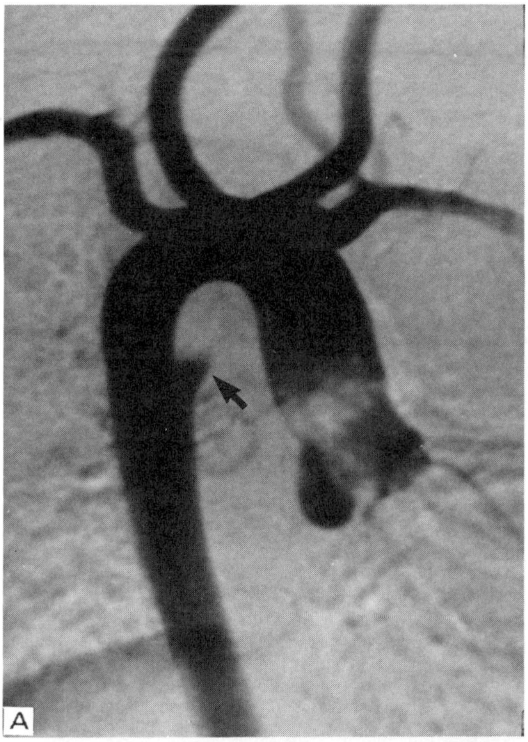

FIGURE 6A. A five-month-old presented with stridor. An esophagogram showed a possible vascular ring. An IADSA demonstrated an unusual aortic arch anomaly. There is a right aortic arch with separate origins of the four brachiocephalic arteries. However, there is a diverticulum from the upper descending thoracic aorta which opacifies with contrast material (arrow) late in imaging.

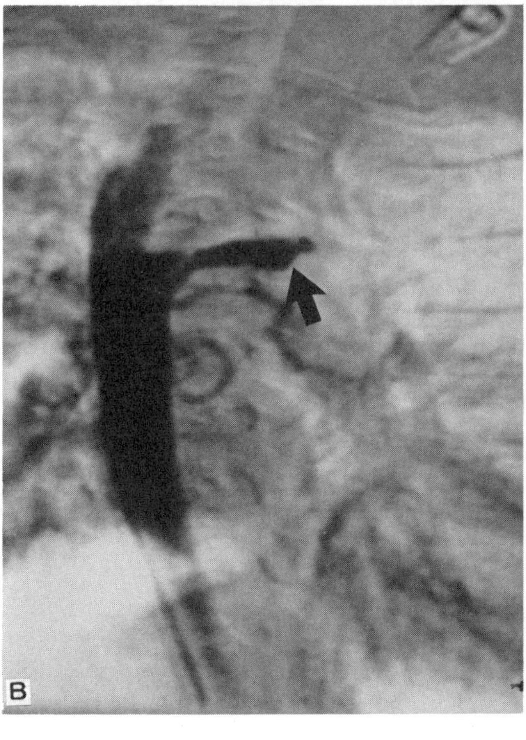

FIGURE 6B. A selective injection into the diverticulum showed patency for approximately 1 cm (arrow). At surgery, the patient was found to have a vascular ring with a ligamentum extending posteriorly from the diverticulum to the pulmonary artery. The vascular ring was successfully ligated at surgery.

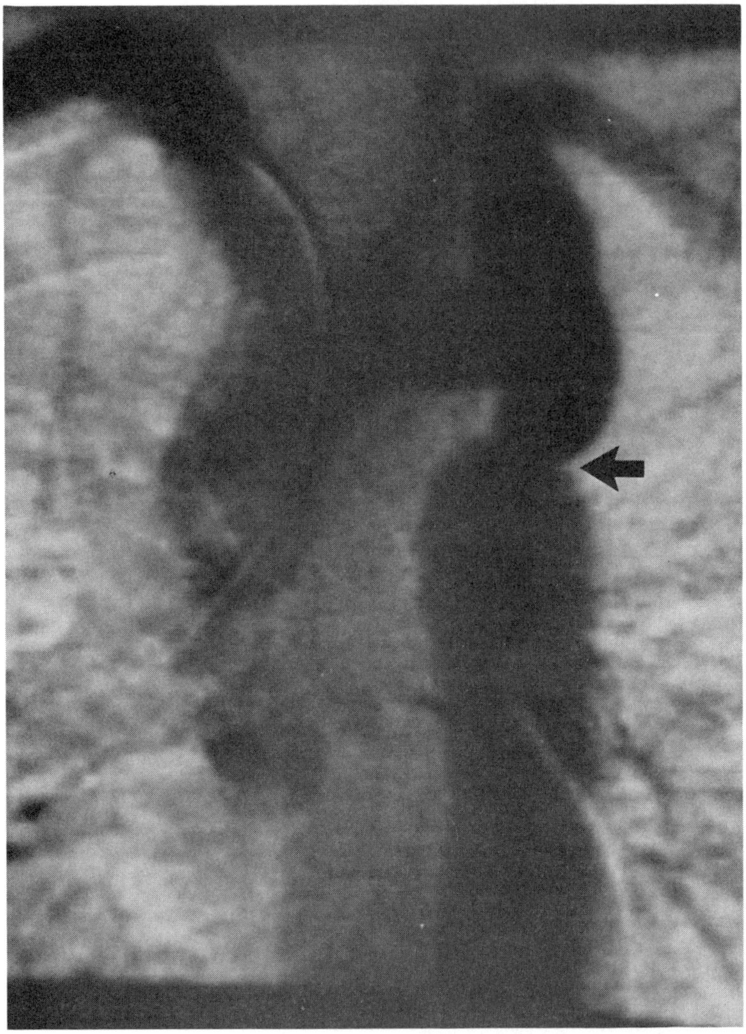

Figure 7. Coarctation of the aorta. A catheter was placed from the right basilic artery into the subclavian artery and into the ascending aorta. An IADSA image was obtained in a slight LAO projection. The study demonstrated dilatation of the left subclavian artery with a tight, discrete coarctation of the aorta (arrow). There is some dilatation of the descending thoracic aorta.

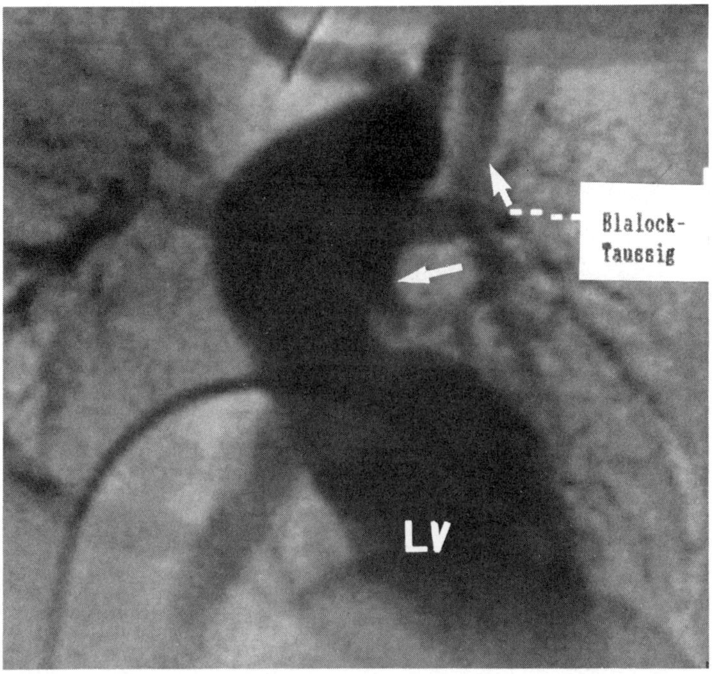

FIGURE 8. Blalock-Taussig shunt. A venous catheter was placed from the inferior vena cava into the right atrium across the atrial septal defect into the left atrium and into the left ventricle (LV). A left ventriculogram demonstrates opacification of the large left-sided aortic arch. There is adequate visualization of the modified left Blalock-Taussig shunt (arrow, Blalock-Taussig). There is opacification of the right pulmonary artery and left pulmonary artery with faint visualization of the main pulmonary artery (arrow). This patient has a hypoplastic right ventricle with an intact ventricular septum and pulmonary atresia.

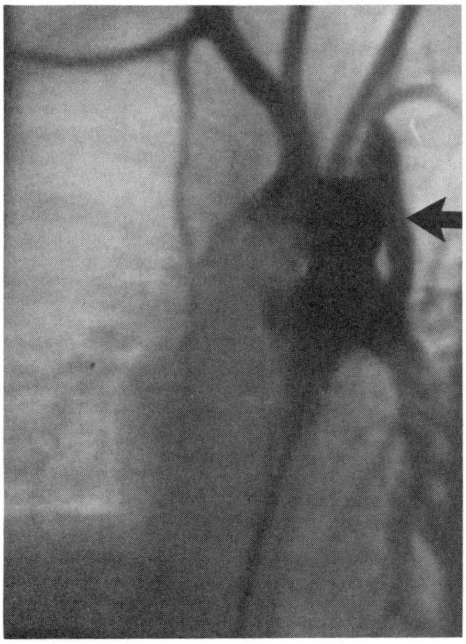

FIGURE 9. Another example of a modified left Blalock-Taussig shunt (arrow) in a patient studied with IADSA. The basic pathology is tricuspid valve atresia and a Glenn procedure has been performed. There is no opacification of the right pulmonary artery from this injection. The Glenn procedure consists of an anastomosis between the superior vena cava and right pulmonary artery. The digital aortogram demonstrated a left aortic arch with normal brachiocephalic vessels. The modified left Blalock-Taussig shunt was easily opacified with filling of the left pulmonary artery in this patient with tricuspid valve atresia.

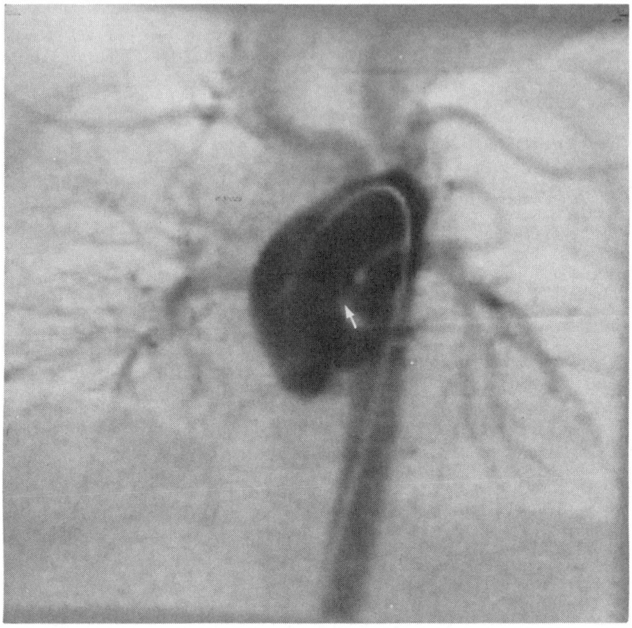

FIGURE 10. IADSA was performed with an aortic injection using cranial angulation. The study showed patency of a central shunt (arrow). The central shunt consists of 4-mm Gortex graft from the ascending aorta to the main pulmonary artery. The basic pathology is that of severe tetralogy of Fallot with pulmonary atresia. The patency of the central shunt allows the pulmonary arteries to grow so that total correction can be performed with a valved conduit in the future.

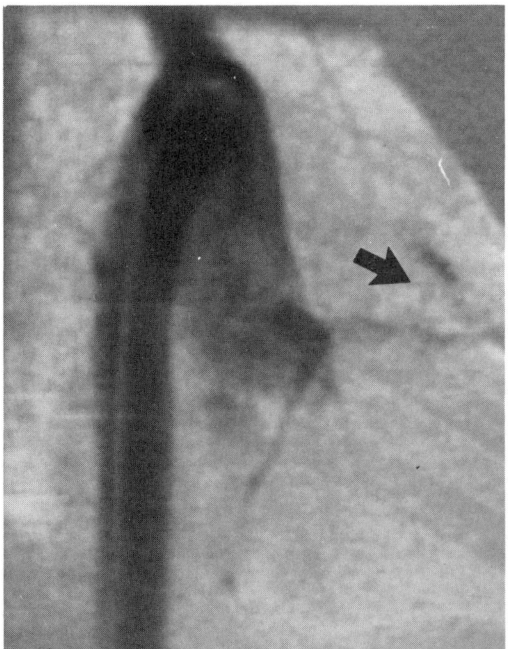

FIGURE 11. Coronary artery fistula. A two-year-old child presented with a continuous murmur. An aortogram in the right anterior oblique projection imaged with IADSA shows a small fistula from the LAD to the left atrium (arrow). This study was imaged with contrast enhancement and a small amount of dilute contrast material using digital imaging techniques. This small fistula was not considered to be a surgical lesion.

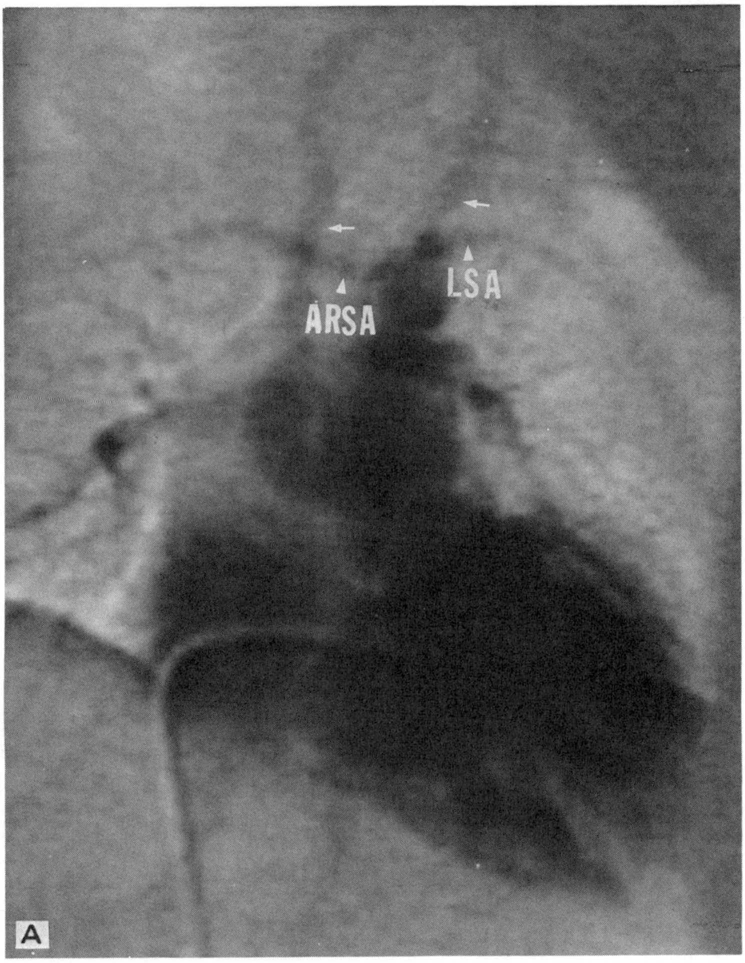

Figure 12A. *A four-day-old infant presented with severe cyanotic congenital heart disease. A right ventriculogram demonstrated a persistent truncus arteriosus with interruption of the aortic arch. Both carotid arteries are opacified (arrows). In addition, the descending thoracic aorta is opacified through the patent ductus arteriosus. The left subclavian artery (arrowhead, LSA) and aberrant right subclavian artery (arrowhead, ARSA) are opacified late in filming.*

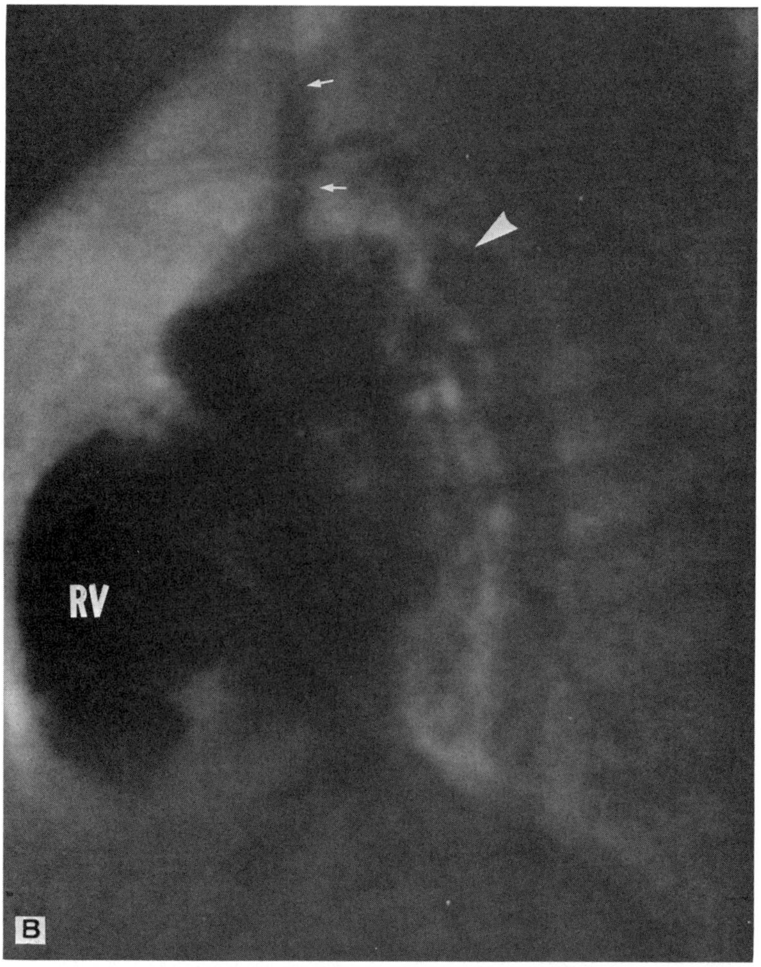

FIGURE 12B. The lateral right ventriculogram (RV) showed a ventricular septal defect and opacification of the left ventricle. There is immediate filling of the persistent truncus arteriosus with both carotid arteries extending cephalad (small arrows). In addition, there is opacification of the descending aorta through the patent ductus arteriosus (arrowhead). This patient developed septic shock and surgical correction could not be performed.

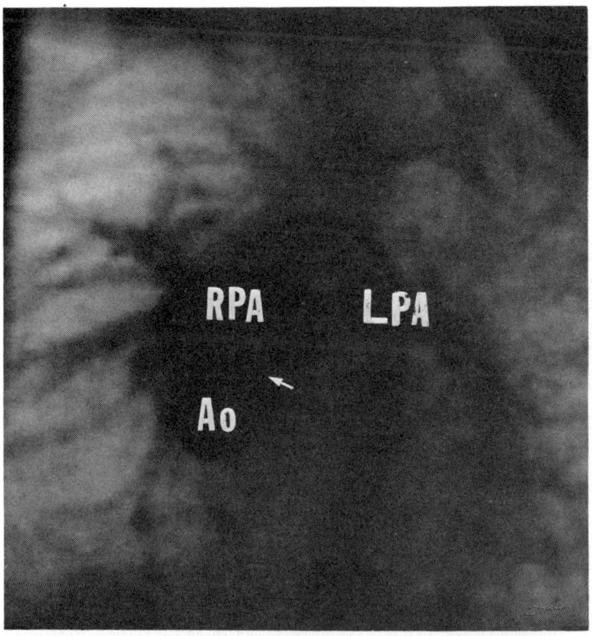

FIGURE 13. Tetralogy of Fallot with aorticopulmonary window. An aortogram was performed with IADSA showing a left-sided aortic arch with an aorticopulmonary window (arrow). There was adequate opacification of both the right pulmonary artery (RPA) and left pulmonary artery (LPA) in this patient with severe tetralogy of Fallot or pulmonary atresia and an aorticopulmonary window. The patient underwent successful correction of this anomaly.

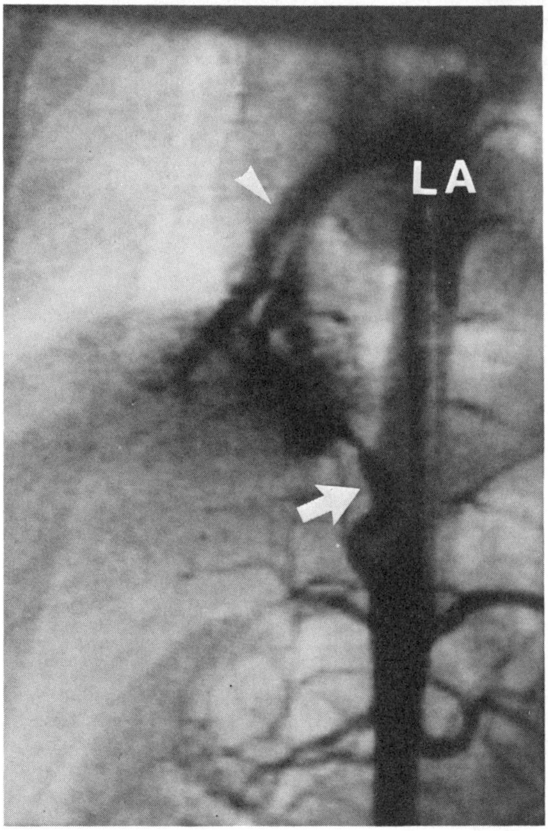

FIGURE 14. Intralobar pulmonary sequestration. An IADSA examination of the lower thoracicoabdominal aorta demonstrated a supplying artery (arrow) arising from the aorta just above the celiac axis. There was opacification of the sequestered segment in the right lower lobe. The pulmonary veins were well imaged (arrowhead) with digital imaging techniques. There was opacification of the lower right pulmonary veins as they enter the left atrium (LA). This lesion was successfully corrected surgically.

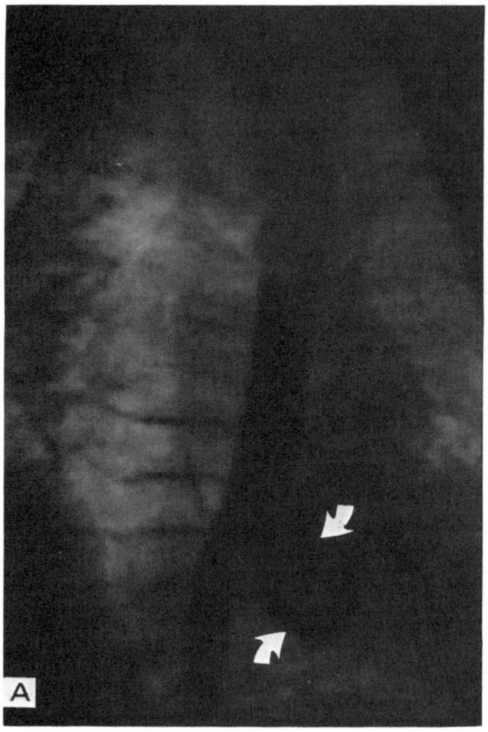

FIGURE 15A. Intrapulmonary sequestration, mixed type. A one-month-old male presented with left lower lobe pneumonia. The IADSA injection into the thoracic aorta demonstrated two supplying arteries to a sequestered segment in the right lower lobe (arrows).

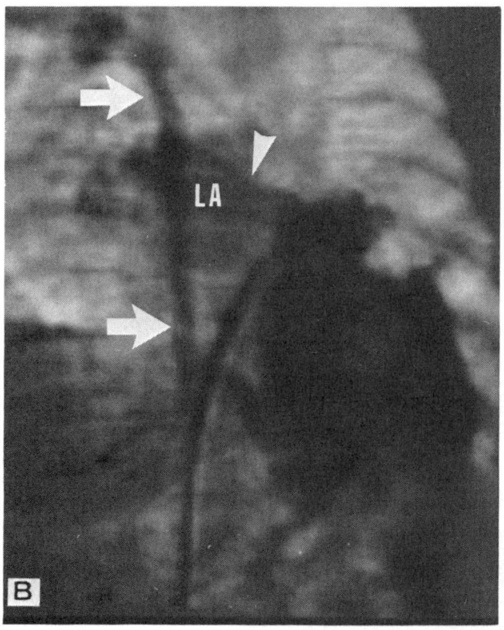

FIGURE 15B. The venous phase or levophase demonstrated dense opacification of the sequestered segment. There is mixed venous drainage with opacification of a left upper pulmonary vein (arrowhead) entering into the left atrium (LA). In addition, there is opacification of the azygous vein (arrows) entering into superior vena cava. This implies both an intralobar component with pulmonary venous return and extralobar component with opacification of azygous or hemiazygous system. This mass was successfully corrected surgically with a thoracicoabdominal approach.

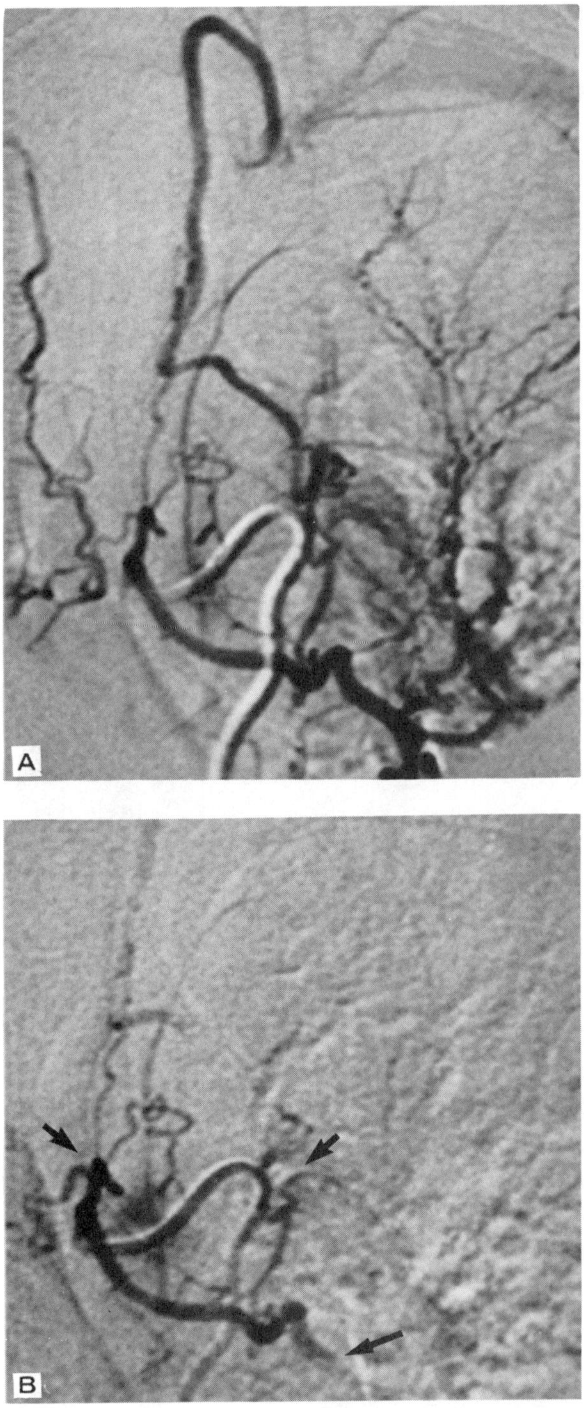

FIGURE 16A,B. ***A:*** *Bronchial embolization for hemoptysis in a 31-year-old female with cystic fibrosis. A left bronchial artery (arrow) was injected with a 6.7F Mikaelsson catheter. IADSA demonstrated large bronchial collaterals to the left upper lobe with areas of extravasation of contrast material due to hemorrhage.* ***B:*** *The left upper bronchial artery was embolized with Ivalon and the distal vessels are occluded implying control of hemorrhage (arrows).*

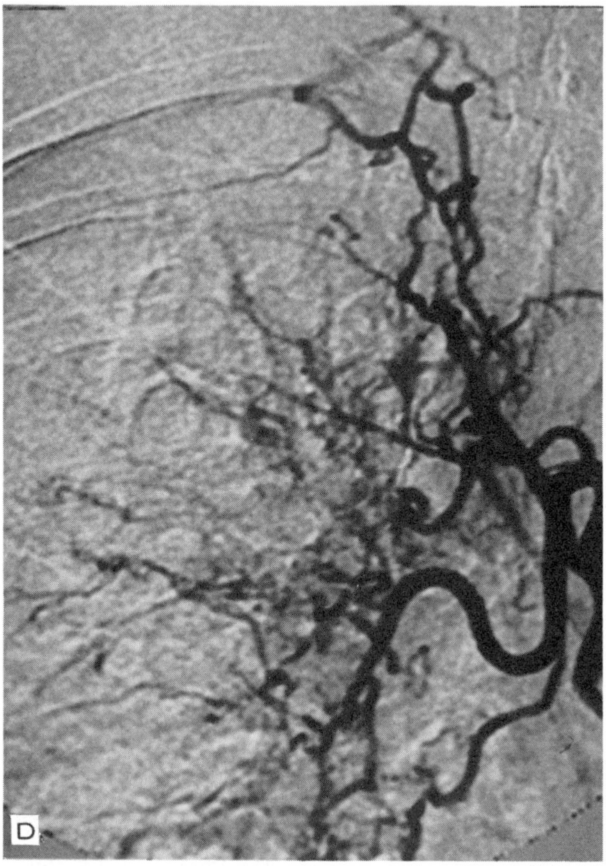

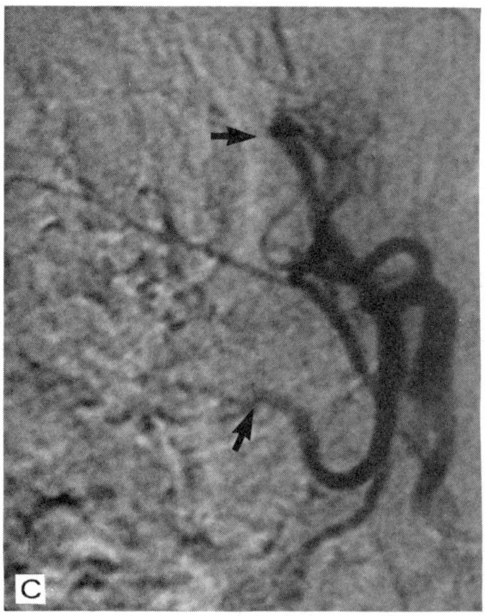

Figure 16C,D. **C:** *An injection into a large right bronchial artery showed extravasation of contrast material in the distal vessels of this patient.* **D:** *The right bronchial artery was also embolized with Ivalon and the hemorrhage was controlled (arrows). IADSA facilitated the interventional procedure, in that images may be visualized immediately in real time. This imaging technique helps prevent embolic complications and a safer, more rapid procedure can be performed with the use of IADSA for interventional procedures.*

References

1. Ovitt T, Capp MP, Christenson P, et al: Development of a digital video subtraction system for intravenous angiography. *SPIE* 206:73–76, 1979.
2. Ovitt TW, Christenson PC, Fisher HD, et al: Intravenous angiography using digital video subtraction: X-ray imaging system. *AJR* 135:1141–1144, 1980.
3. Harrington DP, Boxt LM, Murray PD: Digital subtraction angiography: Overview of technical principles. *AJR* 139:781–786, 1982.
4. Wagner ML, Singleton EB, Egan ME: Digital subtraction angiography in children. *AJR* 140:127–134, 1983.
5. Fletcher BD, Jacobstein MD, Morrison SC: Intravenous digital subtraction angiography (IVDSA) in children. *Pediatr Radiol* 14:425–430, 1984.
6. Tonkin ILD, Fitch SJ, Magill HL, et al: Pediatric digital subtraction angiography: Intraarterial and intracardiac applications. *Pediatr Radiol* 16:126–130, 1986.
7. Faerber EN, Griska LAB, Swartz JD, et al: Digital subtraction angiography in pediatric cerebrovascular occlusive disease. *Radiology* 152:391–394, 1984.
8. Moodie DS, Yiannikas J, Gill CC, et al: Intravenous digital subtraction angiography in the evaluation of congenital abnormalities of the aorta and aortic arch. *Am Heart J* 104:628–634, 1982.
9. Sahn DJ, Valdes-Cruz LM, Ovitt TW, et al: Two dimensional echocardiography and intravenous digital video subtraction angiography for diagnosis and evaluation of double aortic arch. *Am J Cardiol* 50:342–346, 1982.
10. Tonkin IL, Gold RE, Moser D, et al: Evaluation of vascular rings with digital subtraction angiography. *AJR* 142:1287–1291, 1984.
11. Guthaner DF, Miller DC: Digital subtraction angiography of aortic dissection. *AJR* 141:157–161, 1983.
12. Miller FJ, Mineau DE, Koehler PR, et al: Clinical intra-arterial digital subtraction imaging. *Radiology* 148:273–278, 1983.
13. Chang R, Kaufman SL, Kadir S, et al: Digital subtraction angiography in interventional radiology. *AJR* 142:363–366, 1984.
14. Kaufman SL, Chang R, Kadir S, et al: Intraarterial digital subtraction angiography in diagnostic arteriography. *Radiology* 151:323–327, 1984.
15. Tobis JM, Henry WL, Nalcioglu O: Cardiac applications of digital subtraction angiography. *Appl Radiol/Cardiac Imaging* 61–67, 1983.
16. Buonocore E, Pavlicek W, Modic MT, et al: Anatomic and functional imaging of congenital heart disease with digital subtraction angiography. *Radiology* 147:647–654, 1983.
17. Levin AR, Goldberg HL, Borer JS, et al: Digital angiography in the pediatric patient with congenital heart disease: Comparison with standard methods. *Circulation* 68(2):374–384, 1983.
18. Capp MP, Ovitt TW: Digital angiography in the diagnosis of congenital heart disease: An alternative viewpoint. *Cardiovasc Intervent Radiol* 7:190–191, 1984.
19. Tonkin, IL: Digital subtraction angiography in congenital heart disease. *Semin Roentgenol* 20:283–289, 1985.
20. Tonkin ILD, Stapleton FB, Roy S: Digital subtraction angiography in the evaluation of renal vascular hypertension in children *Pediatrics* 81:150–158, 1988.
21. Anthony CL, Tonkin, IL, Marin-Garcia J, et al: A double-blind randomized clinical study of the safety, tolerability, and efficacy of Hexabrix in pediatric angiocardiography. *Invest Radiol* 19(6 Suppl):S335–343, 1984.

Chapter 6

Cerebral Digital Subtraction Angiography

Eric N. Faerber

The advent of newer, noninvasive imaging modalities including ultrasonography, computed tomography, and magnetic resonance imaging has led neuroradiology to new frontiers. The impact of these imaging techniques has been enormous. Although the need for angiography has decreased, there will be specific instances where direct visualization of the intracranial vasculature is required. Digital subtraction angiography (DSA), especially intravenous digital subtraction angiography (IVDSA), is especially appealing for use in infants and children because of its simplicity of technique and associated lower morbidity rate.

Historically, the technique of cerebral angiography was pioneered by Egas Moniz in 1927.[1] He surgically exposed the carotid artery and introduced a needle into the artery under direct visualization. Moniz, however, performed percutaneous procedures as well. Percutaneous techniques were further refined by Loman and Myerson in 1936, using Thorotrast as the contrast agent.[2] Vertebral arterial punctures were performed by Takahashi in 1940.[3] It was not until 1944, however, that the morbidity of angiography was reduced to acceptable levels as a result of angiographic advances made by Engeset.[4] In the 1950s rapid film changing equipment was introduced and has since been significantly improved. Many other improvements and innovations have been introduced, such as mechanical injectors and water soluble contrast media, that have advanced the science of angiography appreciably. A further innovation was the introduction of the Seldinger catheter technique in 1953.[5]

Intravenous angiography was originally described by Robb and Steinberg in 1939.[6] This technique did not gain acceptance because of technical problems in attaining images of good quality. A particular problem was the need to inject large amounts of contrast medium in order to achieve adequate visualization of large arteries and veins. In addition, timing of the circulation was not always successful.

Digital Subtraction Imaging in Infants and Children, edited by Eric N. Faerber. Mount Kisco, New York: Futura Publishing Company, Inc., © 1989.

DSA of the cerebral vasculature developed from the research in digital fluoroscopy which emanated from the University of Arizona,[7] the University of Wisconsin,[8] and the Kiel Kinderklinik in Germany.[9] DSA imaging of the cerebral vasculature was first described by Christenson and co-workers in 1980.[10] Numerous reports soon followed, attesting to the usefulness of this technique.[11–13] There is already a plethora of reports on the widespread usefulness of the intravenous and intra-arterial applications of cerebral DSA in adult patients. The use of this modality in head and neck disease is well established.[14–21] In addition to intracranial applications, there are also increasing indications for the use of DSA in otorhinolaryngology[22,23] and ophthalmology.[24,25] There are relatively few reports of the cerebral applications of DSA in children. However, the technique has successfully displayed a wide spectrum of abnormalities in neonates, infants, and children.[26–31]

Technique

There are a number of factors in the approach to cerebral DSA in infants and children that are essential in order to attain a successful and diagnostic study.

Immobilization

In order to ensure a satisfactory study, limitation of patient movement is essential. Although sophisticated postprocessing techniques are available, patient motion must be kept to a minimum or eliminated during data acquisition.

To immobilize the child's head, the application of tape over the forehead is usually sufficient. In some instances, head clamps may be applied. Recently, a reversible iatrogenic depression of the cranial vault has been described in infants following the use of commercially available head clamps. Newer, fully spongy models of head-holding devices which have large contact surfaces are recommended if head clamps are to be used.[32] A head immobilization technique employing a bite block consisting of a Codman (Codman & Shurtleff, Inc., A Johnson & Johnson Co., Randolph, MA) surgical retractor and sterile tongue blades has been described, although it has not been routinely used in infants and children.[33]

In older children who are able to cooperate, motion artifacts may be reduced by careful instruction to the patient during the study and by the use of low-osmolality contrast media. Other methods used to offset motion artifacts include acquisition of numerous masks prior to injection of contrast medium, the use of rapid frame rates, and pixel shifting.[34]

Sedation and Patient Preparation

Sedation is of paramount importance in addition to immobilization of the child. It is important to note, however, that the newborn infant may not require sedation. The sedation used most frequently in older infants and children for neuroradiologic procedures is oral chloral hydrate (80–100 mg/kg) administered 30 minutes prior to the study. Although there is no single ideal sedative agent, chloral hydrate has the advantages of a wide safety margin and ease of administration.[35] In those children who are refractory to chloral hydrate, intravenous diazepam (0.1 mg/kg) has been used with careful attention to monitoring vital signs. This combination, however, has led to increased agitation in some children. Alternative methods of sedation include an intramuscular preparation of atropine, meperidine, promethazine, and secobarbital (0.08 mL/kg).[35] General anesthesia is seldom required and is used as a last resort in those patients refractory to the above regimens of sedation. Older children generally do not require sedation unless there is emotional instability or mental retardation. A thorough explanation of the procedure to both the older child and his/her parents will aid greatly in allaying their anxieties. Taking the time to give the child and the parents a tour through the angiographic suite, as well as showing and explaining the equipment to them, will also considerably reduce some of the anxiety they may have concerning the impending study.

Oral feeding is generally restricted for four to six hours prior to the study. Adequate hydration must be ensured. Intravenous fluids are routinely administered via a peripheral vein during the study in order to maintain hydration and also to provide open intravenous access when necessary.[28]

Site of Injection

Both intravenous and intra-arterial routes for DSA are now being utilized, with increasing use of intra-arterial DSA in adults.[36–42] Intra-arterial DSA (IADSA) does offer many advantages over conventional angiography such as: immediate image availability with subtraction capability; decreased procedure time and discomfort to the patient; decreased need for selective catheterization; decreased contrast concentration and dose; increased contrast sensitivity; and decreased film cost.[31,43] The advantages of IADSA are certainly most appealing. In infants and children, however, IVDSA is more widely employed. Patient morbidity is considerably reduced by IVDSA when compared to IADSA in which there is a high complication rate associated with femoral arterial punctures in children.[31,44]

For IVDSA, a central venous injection is preferable to an injection in a peripheral vein.[45,46] The catheter is introduced into the femoral vein for inferior vena cava placement or an antecubital vein for superior vena cava placement. In young children, the catheter may be introduced into the external jugular vein.[29]

Catheters

Straight catheters with sideholes are preferable to pigtail catheters. In small children, pigtail catheters are especially painful at insertion and are traumatic to veins.[47] A 3 F or 4 F catheter with sideholes is used in the young child, whereas a 5 F catheter with sideholes is more appropriate for older children. It is important to note that the largest catheter deemed suitable for central venous placement should be used in order to facilitate delivery of the contrast bolus.[48]

Contrast Medium and Flow Rate

The contrast media we use for IVDSA is Renografin 60 or Renografin 76 (E.R. Squibb & Sons, Inc., Princeton, NJ). The volume of contrast medium administered for each "run" is 1 mL/kg of body weight with a maximum volume of 4 mL/kg of body weight/study.[28] The concentration of the contrast medium, however, may be diluted to a 45% solution.[49] The flow rate used is 6–15 mL/sec through a catheter placed in the inferior vena cava.

Two new groups of contrast media offer great potential for DSA. In the first group are ionic, dimeric, contrast media. Hexabrix (ioxaglate meglumine 39.3% and ioxaglate sodium 19.6%, 320 mg/mL iodine) (Mallinckrodt, Inc., St. Louis, MO) contains double the number of iodine molecules within the anionic portion of the molecule as compared with monomeric ionic contrast media of the same osmolality. Patients who have had Hexabrix injected into an external carotid artery experienced less warmth or burning sensations, which has resulted in less patient motion.[31] This decrease in patient discomfort is attributed to the reduced osmolality of this contrast agent.[50]

In the second group of newer contrast media, are nonionic monomeric agents which include iopamidol (Isovue, Squibb) and iohexol (Omnipaque, Winthrop Laboratories, New York, NY). In this group, the sodium or meglumine cations have been replaced by side chains which do not dissociate from the iodine containing portion of the molecule. It is this property, as well as the tendency of the molecules to aggregate in solution, which leads to the markedly lower osmolality of this group as compared with current ionic angiographic contrast media.[50]

Radiographic Projections

The two most useful projections for cerebral DSA are the Towne and frontal views. Side-to-side comparison of the intracranial vasculature can be readily made when these projections are used (Fig. 1). The lateral projection is of limited use because in this projection there is significant superimposition of vessels. The lateral projection, however, may be useful in demonstrating suprasellar lesions and in the evaluation of veins and dural sinuses (Fig. 2).[31]

Oblique projections of the intracranial vasculature have been tried in order to offset the superimposition of arteries that occur with lateral projections, but these have not proved to be of particular value in achieving the desired result. The venous sinuses, however, are demonstrated on oblique as well as frontal and lateral projections (Fig. 3). Oblique projections of the neck have proved more useful in the evaluation of the carotid bifurcation and proximal arterial obstructions (Fig. 4). In addition, oblique projections of the aorta and origin of the great vessels can be conveniently obtained during the examination (Fig. 5).

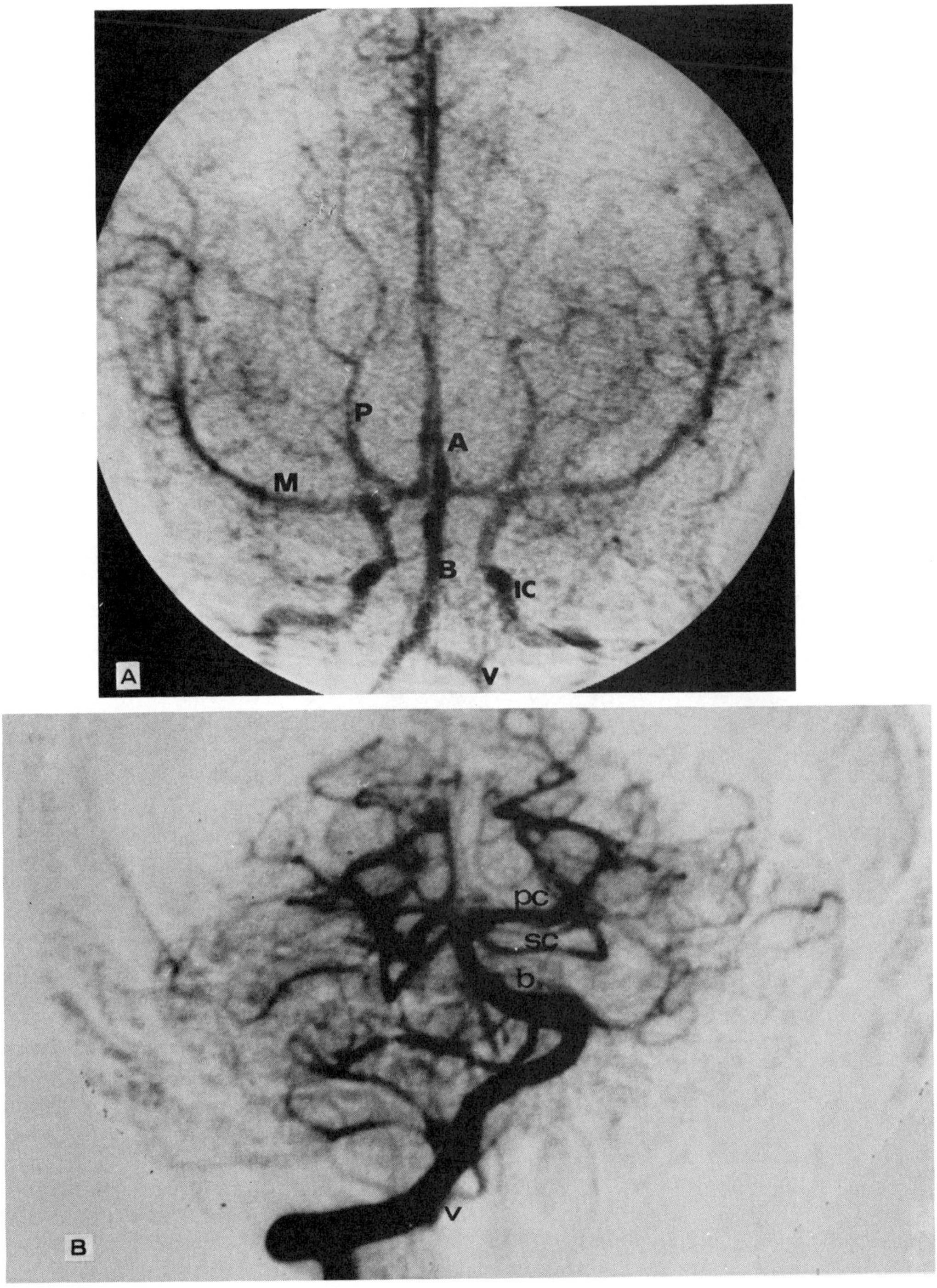

FIGURE 1. ***A***: *IVDSA frontal projection. A = anterior cerebral artery; B = basilar artery; IC = internal carotid artery; M = middle cerebral artery; P = posterior cerebral artery; V = vertebral artery.* ***B***: *IADSA frontal projection. Selective vertebral injection demonstrating vertebral artery (v), basilar artery (b), superior cerebellar artery (sc), posterior cerebral artery (pc).*

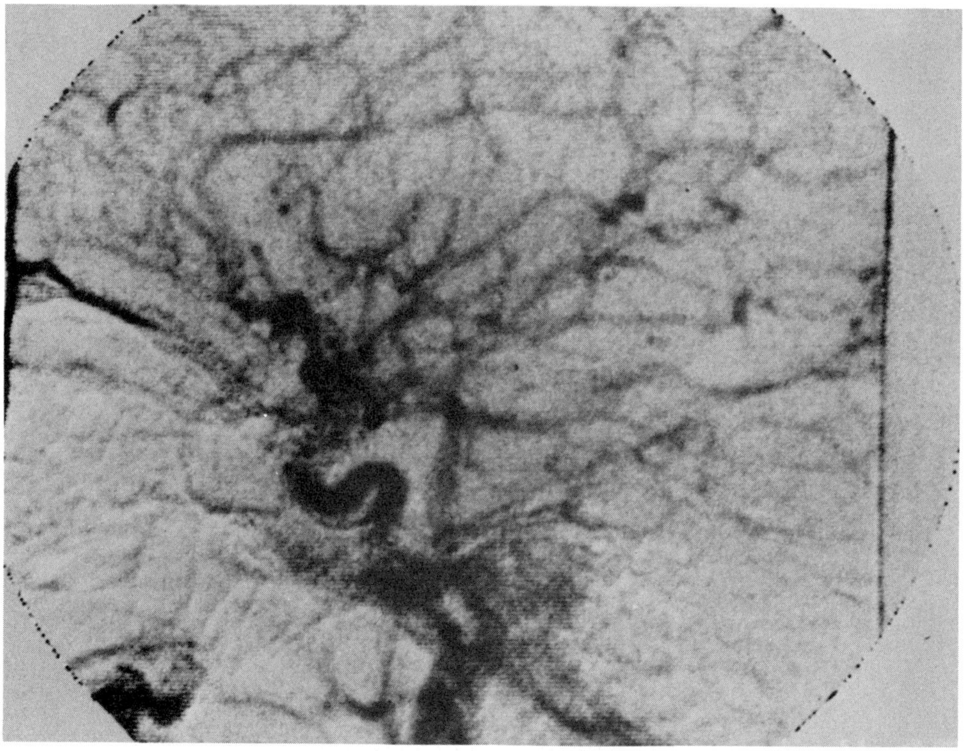

FIGURE 2. *IVDSA lateral projection. There is overlap of vessels, but this projection is useful for demonstration of suprasellar lesions.*

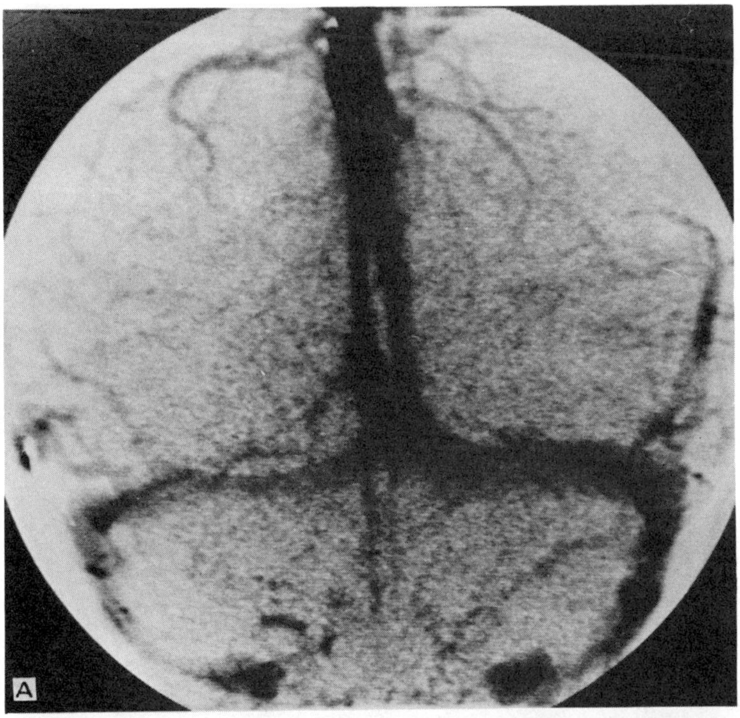

FIGURE 3A. *IVDSA frontal projection demonstrates venous sinuses.*

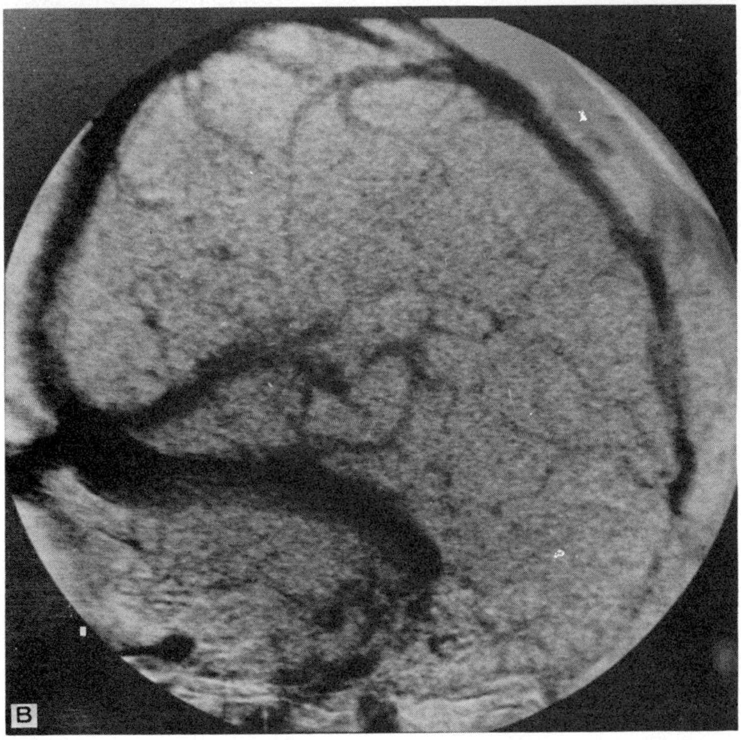

FIGURE 3B. *IVDSA oblique projection demonstrates venous sinuses.*

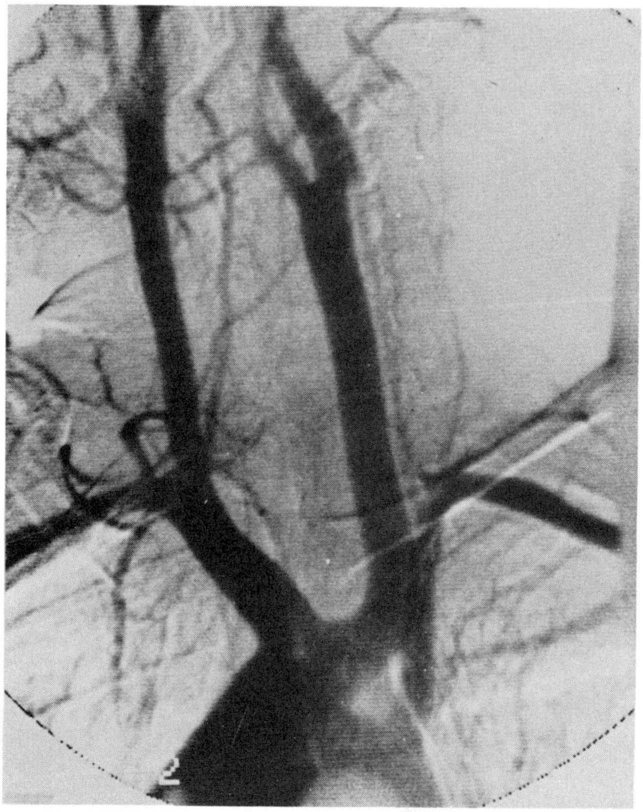

Figure 4. Right posterior oblique projection IVDSA demonstrates the common carotid arteries, carotid bifurcations, and vertebral arteries.

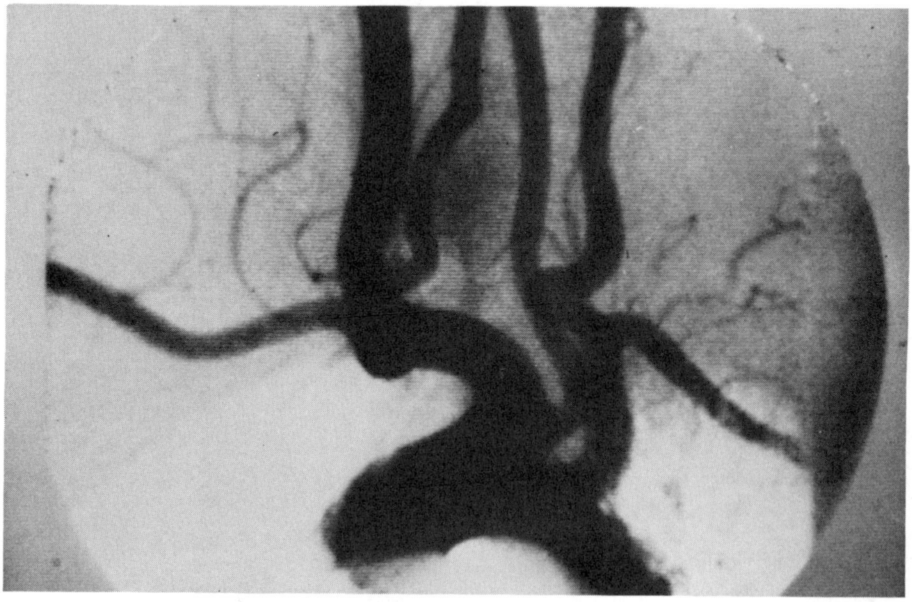

Figure 5. IVDSA of aortic arch demonstrates the origin of the great vessels.

This projection is of value in the evaluation of patients with arteritis and collagen vascular disorders.

Applications of Cerebral DSA

Although there are few reports attesting to the usefulness of this technique in infants and children, a number of appropriate indications exist for the application of cerebral DSA in the pediatric age group.

Preoperative Demonstration of Arterial Vasculature

The advent of newer imaging modalities has led to a decline in the number of cerebral angiograms performed in children. Nonetheless, preoperative arterial vascular mapping may often be required by the neurosurgeons in planning the surgical approach to supratentorial tumors and, occasionally, infratentorial tumors.

Aneurysms

Cerebral aneurysms are less frequently encountered in infants and children than they are in adults. In some instances, the presence of single or multiple aneurysms may elude neuroradiologic demonstration. In order to successfully demonstrate an aneurysm, multiple injections of a single artery in different projections may be required.[51]

IVDSA in combination with high-resolution CT may be used successfully in screening for aneurysms as a cause of symptoms in patients with specific cranial nerve palsy.[52] Although IVDSA is useful in screening for a suspected aneurysm demonstrated on CT, it is not the definitive study for the evaluation of intracranial aneurysms. IVDSA has a relatively poor spatial resolution, as well as the added problems of vessel overlap on lateral and oblique projections and misregistration artifacts. Large aneurysms can readily be detected by IVDSA; however, small aneurysms may be missed. Aneurysms are especially apt to be missed if their diameter is less than twice that of the parent artery.[53] The neck of an aneurysm is poorly delineated by IVDSA. In order to accurately define the neck of an aneurysm, conventional angiography is usually necessary.[50–54] Postoperatively, IVDSA is useful in demonstrating the successful ligation of the aneurysm.[55]

Another important use of IVDSA is in the documentation and evaluation of cerebral vasospasm following acute rupture of an aneurysm.[55,56] The attenuation of the arterial caliber of one cerebral hemisphere (unilateral vasospasm) or generalized poor visualization of all intracranial vessels (diffuse vasospasm) is readily observed by means of cerebral IVDSA.[55]

Vascular Malformations

IVDSA is a useful screening technique for the confirmation of vascular malformations demonstrated on CT (Fig. 6). The sensitivity and specificity of IVDSA in the demonstration of vascular malformations is superior to that of CT.[57] However, both techniques are complementary in the screening of vascular malformations as CT will also provide information with regard to ventricular size, intracerebral hematoma, and local atrophy.[58] A limitation of IVDSA, however, is the simultaneous opacification of all intracranial arteries and thus the individual vessels to the lesion are less easily delineated. IVDSA is also useful for the postoperative evaluation of the surgical resection or the embolization of a vascular malformation.[18,56]

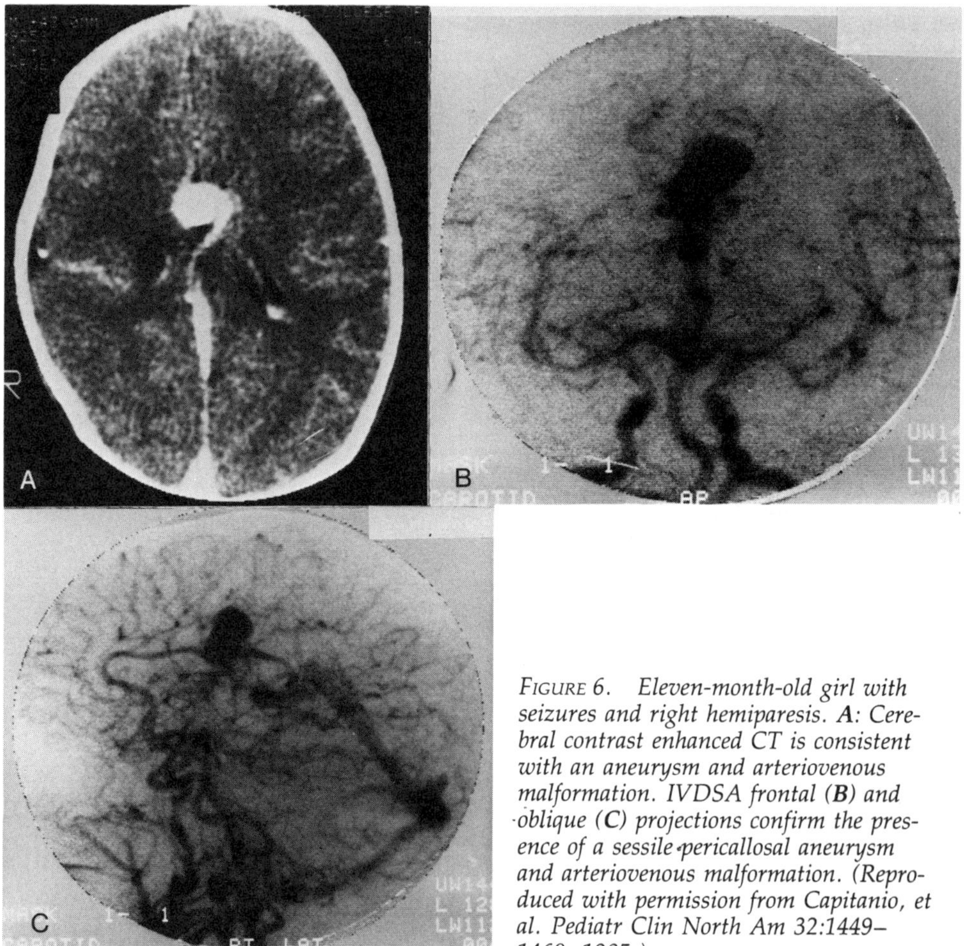

*FIGURE 6. Eleven-month-old girl with seizures and right hemiparesis. **A**: Cerebral contrast enhanced CT is consistent with an aneurysm and arteriovenous malformation. IVDSA frontal (**B**) and oblique (**C**) projections confirm the presence of a sessile pericallosal aneurysm and arteriovenous malformation. (Reproduced with permission from Capitanio, et al. Pediatr Clin North Am 32:1449–1460, 1985.)*

Venous Abnormalities

Dural venous sinuses are well demonstrated by IVDSA. In fact, the dural sinuses are better visualized by IVDSA than by a selective injection of a single carotid artery during conventional angiography. When selective arteriography is performed, a mixture of both nonopacified and opacified blood from each hemisphere is received by the dural venous sinuses. This often results in poor visualization of the sinuses and streaming artifacts.[59] With IVDSA, there is simultaneous opacification of all the intracranial arteries resulting in better visualization of the dural venous sinuses.[59,60] Thus IVDSA is considered to be the preferred method of diagnosing venous sinus occlusion.[59] In infants and children with possible pseudotumor cerebri, IVDSA is therefore an excellent screening modality for exclusion of venous sinus occlusion.

Evaluation of small intracerebral veins is also possible by means of IVDSA. The internal cerebral veins are well seen in the lateral projection, thus thrombosis or displacement of the veins by masses and hydrocephalus are readily demonstrated by IVDSA.[60,61]

Major Arterial Occlusive Disease

Cerebrovascular occlusive disease in infants and children may be due to a wide spectrum of diseases which include: hematologic disorders, diabetes mellitus, autoimmune disorders, neoplasia, congenital heart disease, aneurysms and arteriovenous disorders, homocystinuria, dehydration, and trauma. In some instances the etiology remains obscure.[62]

The decreased spatial resolution of DSA limits visualization of the entire intracranial arterial system. However, we have found this modality to be useful in documenting major occlusive disease in some forms of cerebrovascular occlusive disease.[28] The association of sickle cell disease and cerebral infarction is well established.[63] There had been a reluctance to perform cerebral angiography in patients with sickle cell disease because of the possibility of further sickling following the administration of contrast medium.[64] Angiography is now considered relatively safe provided the patient is well hydrated and has a circulating hemoglobin S concentration of $<20\%$. We have had no complications with this regimen in our cerebral DSA studies in children with sickle cell disease.[28] Large vessel stenoses, vascular occlusions, and collateral circulation are common but nonspecific features of sickle cell disease (Figs. 7–10).

Brain Death

The most reliable confirmatory criterion of brain death is cessation of intracerebral blood flow. This can be demonstrated by selective arteriography which is time consuming, or by radionuclide brain scanning in which it may be difficult to differentiate intracerebral from extracerebral vessels.[65,66] IVDSA en-

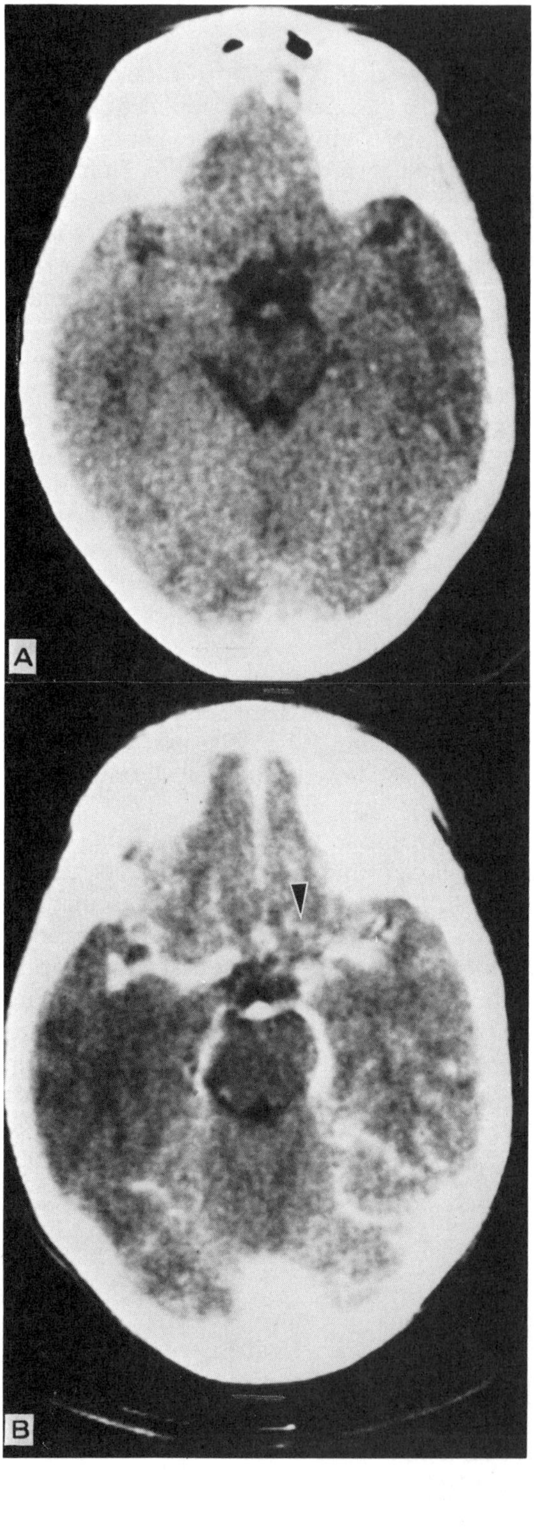

Figure 7. One-year-old boy with sickle cell disease. ***A****: Noncontrast cerebral CT.* ***B****: Contrast enhanced cerebral CT scan demonstrates occlusion of the left internal carotid artery (arrowhead).* ***C****: IVDSA oblique projection reveals occlusion of the left internal carotid artery above the bifurcation (arrowheads).* ***D****: IVDSA frontal projection demonstrates occlusion of the intracranial portion of the left internal carotid artery (arrowheads). (Reproduced with permission from Faerber, et al. Radiology 152:391–394, 1984.)*

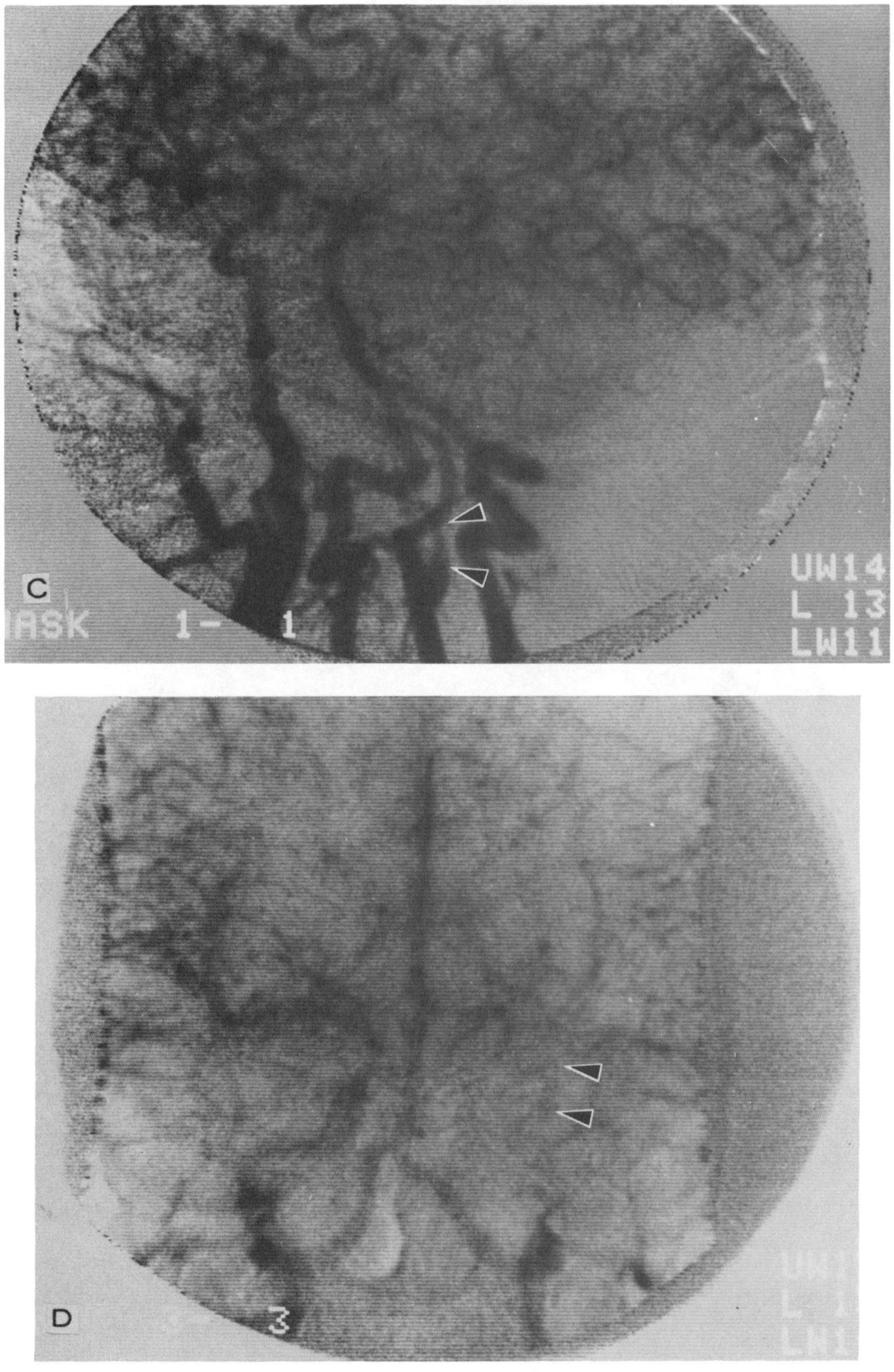

Figures 7C, D.

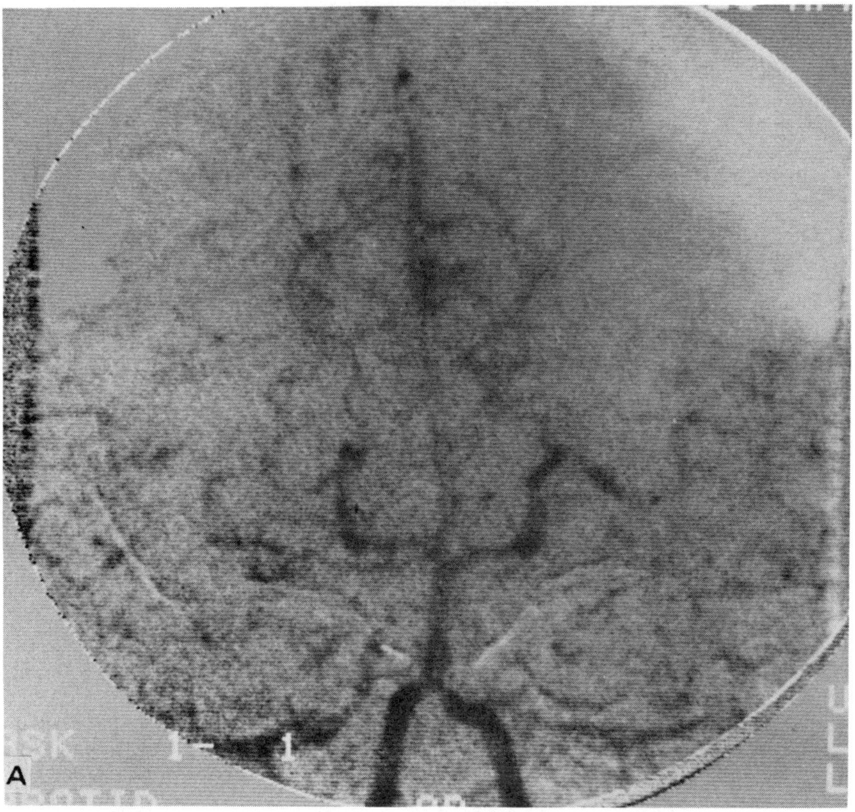

FIGURE 8. Seven-year-old girl with hemiplegia of unknown etiology. ***A****: IVDSA frontal projection demonstrates occlusion of the left internal carotid artery.* ***B****: IVDSA lateral projection reveals occlusion of the left internal carotid artery and filling of the vertebrobasilar system.* ***C****: IVDSA lateral projection (later phase) demonstrates retrograde filling of the anterior and middle cerebral arteries. Reproduced with permission from Faerber et al. Radiology 152:391–394, 1984.*

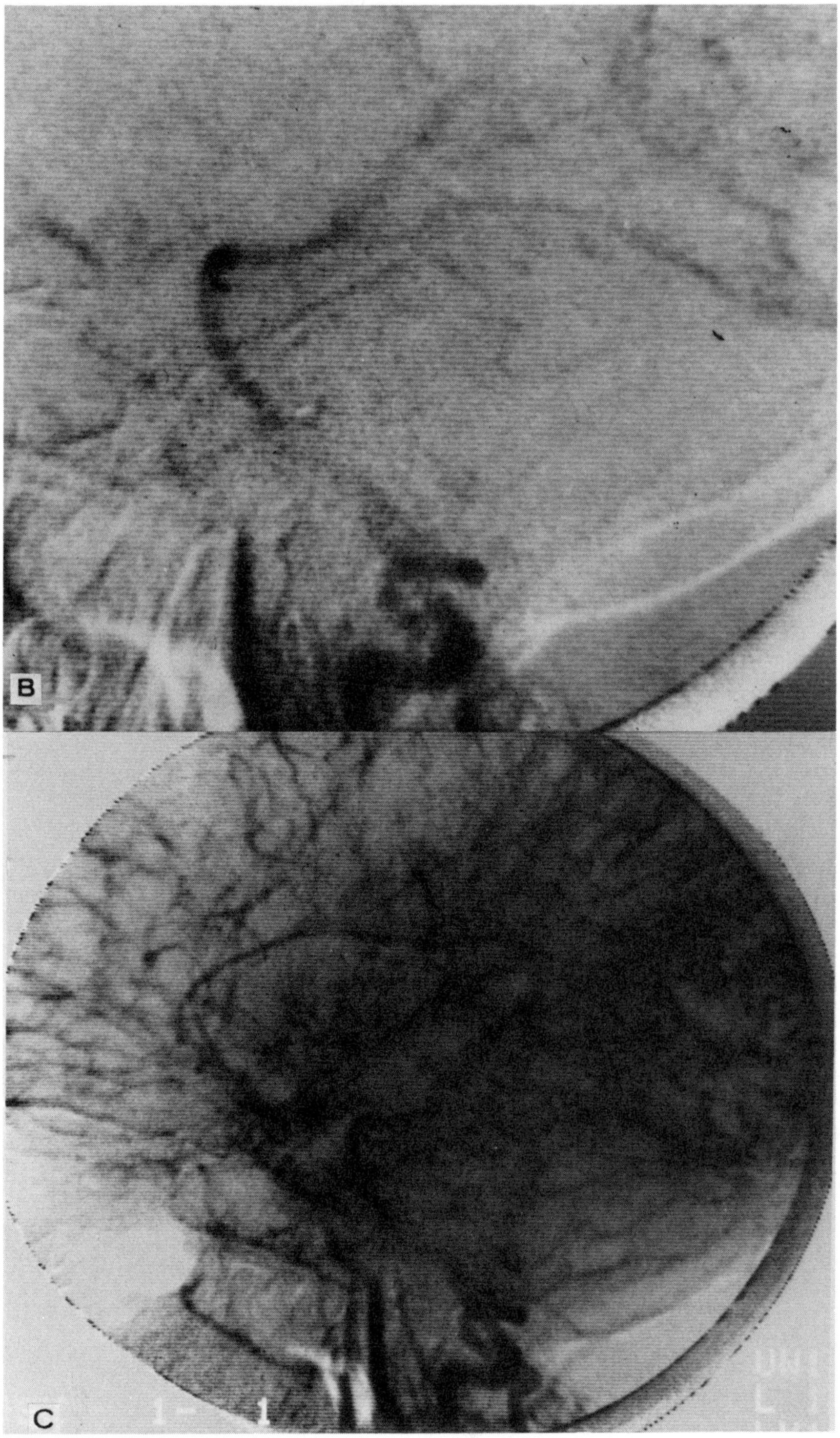

FIGURES 8B, C.

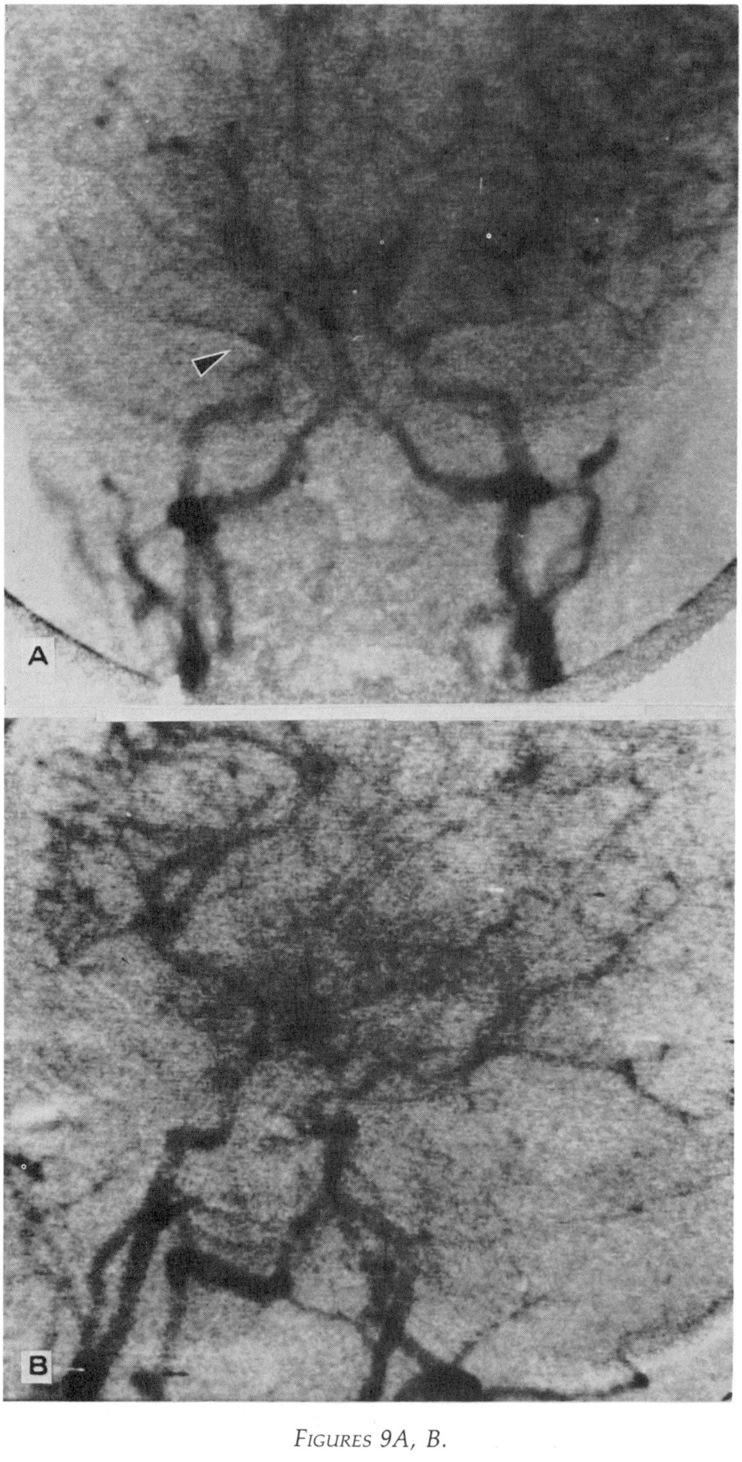

FIGURES 9A, B.

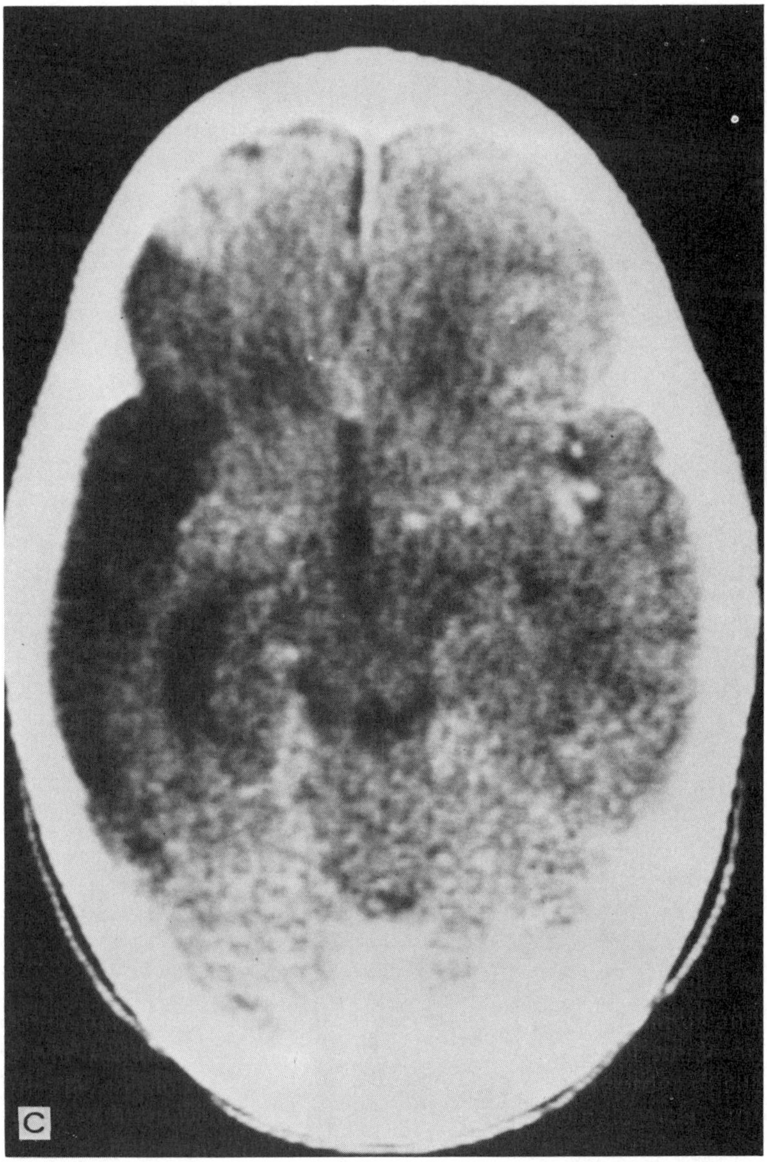

FIGURE 9. *Four-year-old girl with sickle cell disease. **A**: DSA frontal projection. Occlusion of the right middle cerebral artery (arrowhead). **B**: DSA oblique projection. Note Moya-Moya circulation. **C**: Contrast-enhanced head CT demonstrates infarction in the right middle cerebral artery distribution. (Reproduced with permission from Faerber, et al. Radiology 152:391–394, 1984.)*

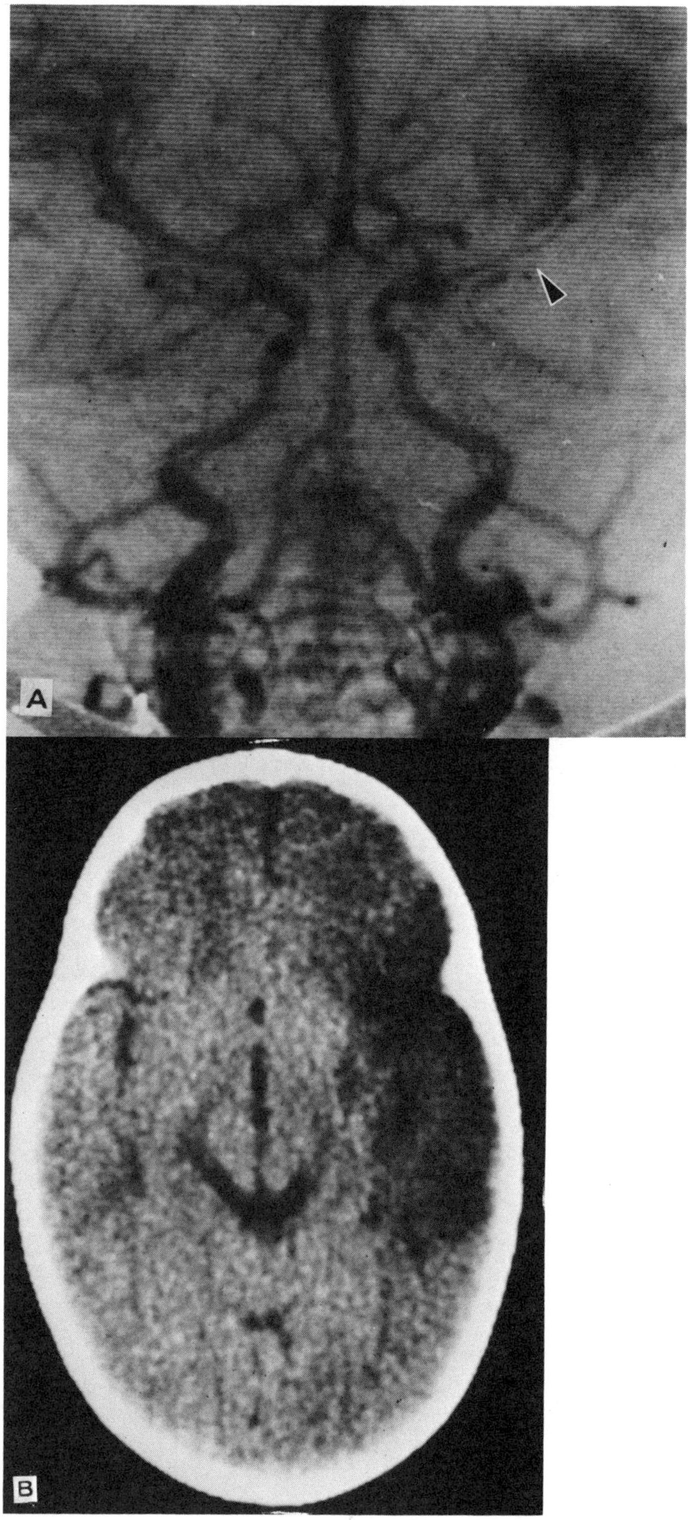

Figure 10. Eighteen-month-old girl with microangiopathic hemolysis and thrombocytopenia. ***A***: *Non-contrast cerebral CT scan demonstrates infarction in the distribution of the left middle cerebral artery.* ***B***: *IVDSA frontal projection demonstrates partial occlusion of the left middle cerebral artery (arrowhead).* ***C***: *IVDSA frontal projection (four months later) reveals progressive occlusion of the left middle cerebral artery.* ***D***: *IVDSA frontal projection (three months after C) demonstrates progressive occlusion of the anterior and middle cerebral arteries and the left posterior cerebral artery. (Reproduced with permission from Faerber, et al. Radiology 152:391–394, 1984.)*

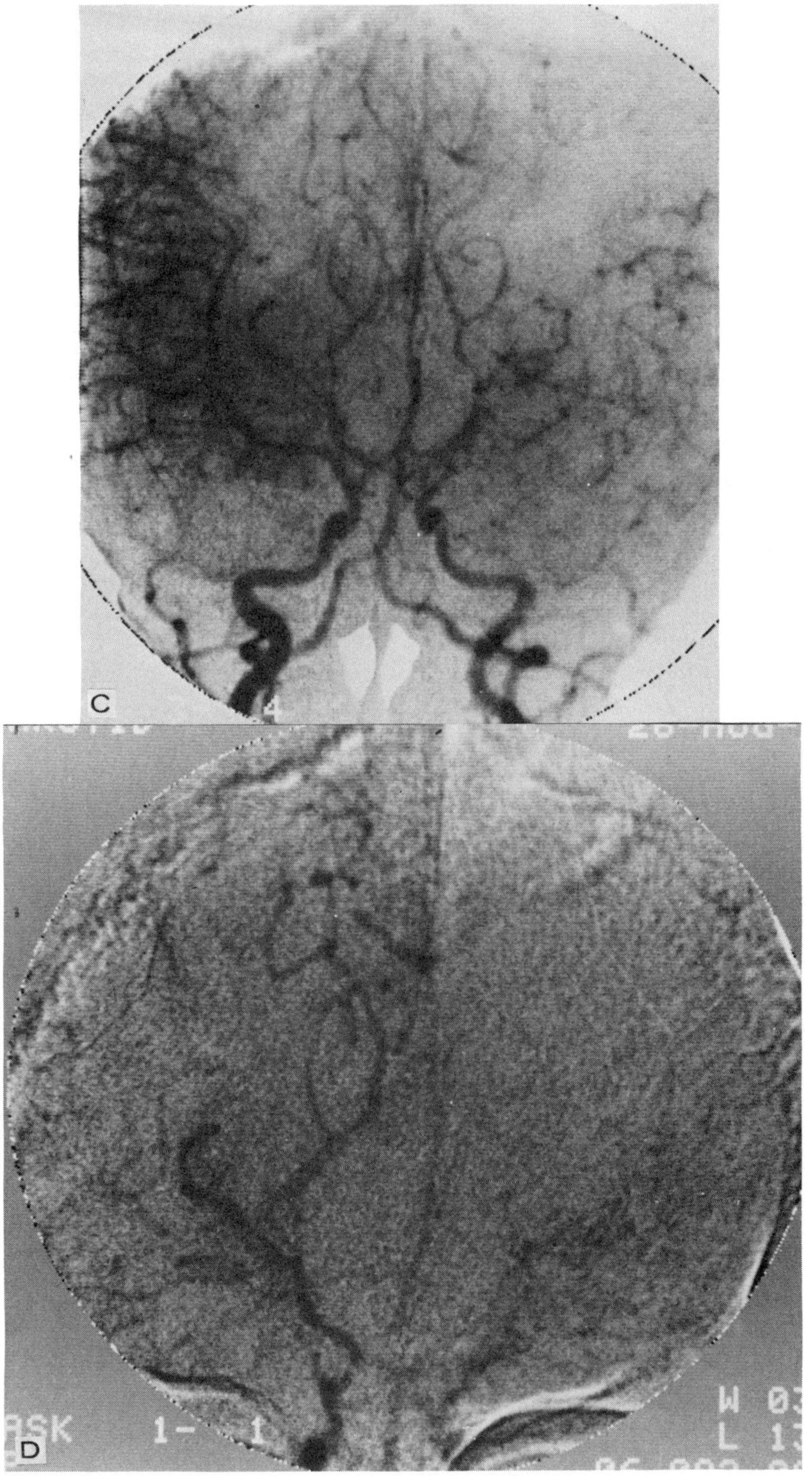

Figures 10C, D.

ables rapid assessment of the status of intracerebral perfusion and permits accurate distinction between intracranial and extracranial vessels.[67] This modality has been used for the diagnosis of brain death in both children and adults.[31,67] Organs planned for transplantation can be examined by the same DSA procedure using either the intravenous or the intra-arterial route.[68]

Tumors

IVDSA is of limited value in the evaluation of intracranial mass lesions. However, this modality is used to provide a "road map" prior to surgery for some tumors such as pituitary tumors and meningiomas.[69] As noted above DSA is of particular value in the preoperative evaluation of sellar and juxtasellar lesions shown on CT, especially in its ability to distinguish between tumor and aneurysm[69,70] (Fig. 11). The limited spatial resolution of IVDSA is inadequate for the demonstration of neovascularity or small arteriovenous shunts encountered in some intracranial tumors.[70] The advantages of improved resolution and the need for small amounts of contrast medium afforded by IADSA make this a suitable technique for the evaluation of mass lesions. However, IADSA is equally invasive as conventional angiography.[70]

Trauma

Cerebral CT is the modality of choice for the evaluation of subsequent management of intracranial lesions secondary to trauma. A chronic subdural hematoma may be an incidental finding in the DSA study of other intracranial lesions. IVDSA, however, is most useful in the evaluation of trauma to the extracranial cervical vasculature (See Chapter 8).

Advantages

IVDSA

1. ease and simplicity in performing study
2. decreased patient morbidity and discomfort
3. study can be performed on an outpatient basis
4. reduced costs
5. total vascular opacification obviates need for selective angiography
6. intravenous method is particularly appealing in infants and children as damage to femoral artery is avoided
7. high contrast resolution
8. radiation exposure less than conventional techniques

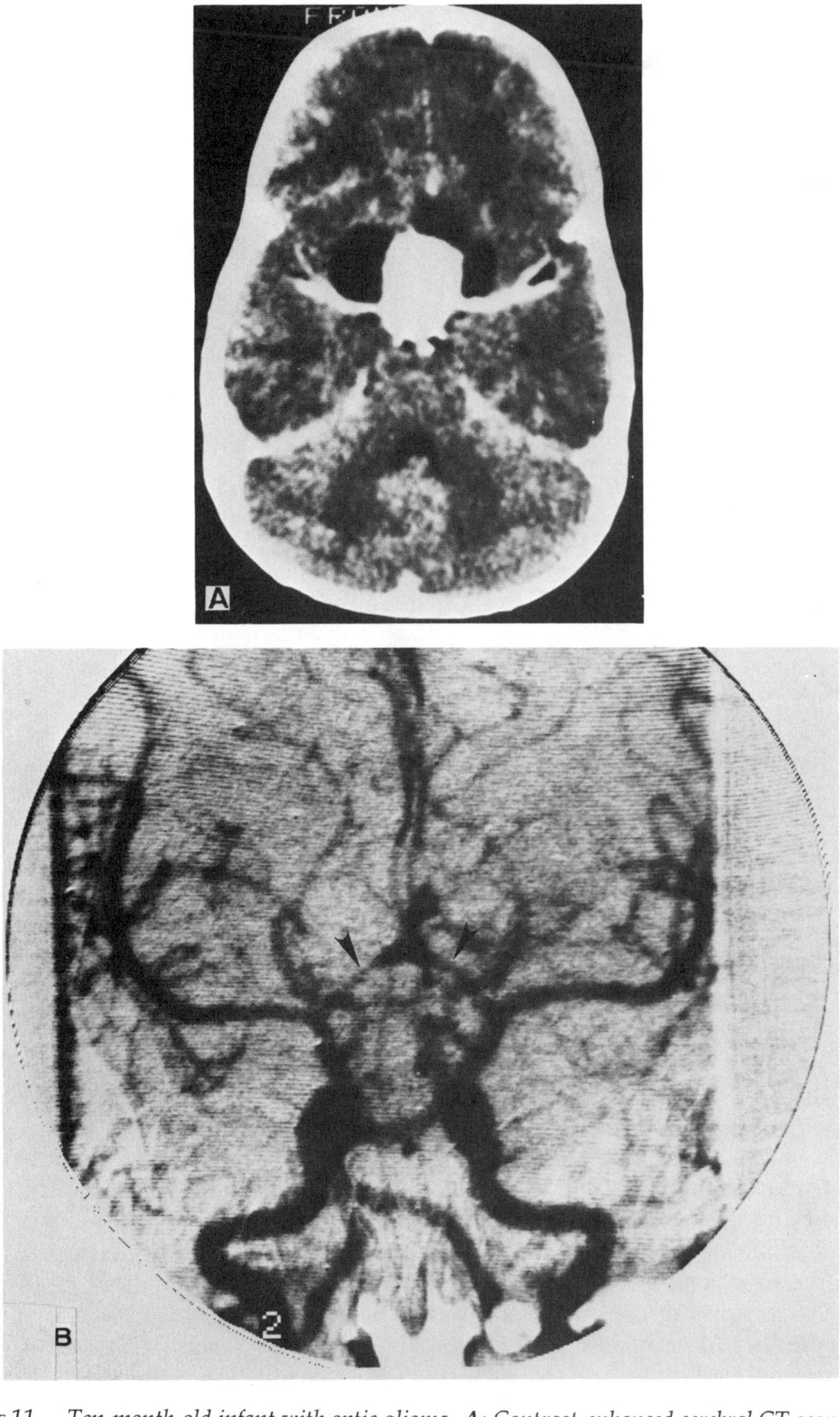

FIGURE 11. *Ten-month-old infant with optic glioma.* ***A****: Contrast-enhanced cerebral CT scan demonstrates an enhancing suprasellar mass.* ***B****: IVDSA frontal projection excludes an aneurysm and demonstrates elevation of the A1 portions of the anterior cerebral arteries (arrowheads) due to the tumor. (Reproduced with permission from Capitanio, et al. Pediatr Clin North Am 32:1449–1460, 1985.)*

IADSA

1. small volume of dilute contrast required
2. less time consuming as electronic subtraction instantly available
3. decreased patient discomfort
4. adequate spatial resolution
5. reduced cost—less film used than conventional angiography

Disadvantages

IVDSA

1. image degradation due to patient motion
2. limited field of view
3. decreased spatial resolution
4. misregistration artifacts
5. large volume of contrast medium required

IADSA

1. femoral arterial damage
2. motion artifacts

Complications

Complications resulting from DSA may be classified into three categories: *local, systemic* and *neurologic*.

Local

Hematoma at the site of catheter insertion may occur with either intravenous or intra-arterial techniques. Use of straight catheters will be less painful to the patient and the incidence of hematoma formation is minimal.

Arterial damage is a potential hazard related to femoral arterial puncture and thus the intravenous route is being adopted for use in infants and children.[31]

Extravasation of contrast medium has been described with the use of short, single end-hold catheters. This complication can be obviated with the use of straight multiside-hole catheters which greatly diminish catheter recoil. Injection rates of 15 mL/sec or less, as well as setting a linear rate rise on the angiographic power injector, will also reduce the recoil.[71]

Focal cellulitis developing at the puncture site is an infrequent complication.[71]

Systemic

Adverse systemic reactions following intravenous administration of iodinated contrast medium generally occurs less frequently in infants and children than in adults. In our series of IVDSA studies we have not encountered complications such as hives, itching, periorbital edema, nasal congestion, or sneezing. Such systemic reactions, however, are commonly encountered in adults following these procedures.[72] Chest pain, acute shortness of breath, hypotension, and pulmonary edema have also been described in adult patients. Transient renal failure due to dehydration of the patient and/or use of excessive volumes of contrast medium have been reported.[46]

Neurologic

Neurologic complications reported in adults following IVDSA occur in 0.5% of cases and have varied from syncope, headache to seizures, and hemiparesis.[72] Neurologic complications in infants and children following DSA procedures have not as yet been reported.

References

1. Moniz E: L'encephalographic arterielle, son importance dans la localisation des tumeurs cerebrales. *Rev Neurol* (Paris) 2:27, 1927.
2. Loman J, Myerson A: Visualization of the cerebral vessels by direct carotid injection of Thorium dioxide (Thoratrast). *Am J Roentgenol Radium Ther* 35:188–193, 1936.
3. Takahashi K: Die percutane arteriographic der arterio vertebralis and ihre versorgungsgebiete. *Arch Psychiat* 111:373–379, 1940.
4. Engeset A: Cerebral angiography with perabrodil. *Acta Radiol* (Stockholm) (Suppl) 56, 1944.
5. Seldinger GI: Catheter replacement of the needle in percutaneous arteriography: A new technique. *Acta Radiol* 39:368–376, 1953.
6. Robb GP, Steinberg I: Visualization of the chambers of the heart, the pulmonary circulation and the great blood vessels in man. A practical method. *Am J Roentgenol Radium Ther* 41:1–17, 1939.
7. Ovitt TW, Capp MP, Fischer HD: The development of a digital video subtraction system for intravenous angiography. *Proc Spie* 167:61, 1978.
8. Kruger RA, Mistretta CA, Lancaster J, et al: A digital video image processor for real time subtraction imaging. *Opt Eng* 17:652–657, 1978.
9. Brennecke R, Brown TK, Bursch J, et al: Computerized video-image processing with application to cardioangiographic roentgen image series. In Nagel HH (Ed): *Digital Image Processing*. New York, Springer-Verlag, 1977.
10. Christenson PC, Ovitt TW, Fisher HD III, et al: Intravenous angiography using digital video subtraction: Intravenous cervacocerebrovascular angiography. *AJNR* 1:379–386, 1980.
11. Chilcote WA, Modic MT, Pavlicker WA, et al: Digital subtraction angiography of the carotid arteries. A comparative study in 100 patients. *Radiology* 139:287–295, 1981.
12. Carmody RF, Smith JRL, Seeger JF, et al: Intravenous cerebral angiography: Early clinical experience. *Ariz Med* 38:349–350, 1981.

13. Little JR, Furlan AJ, Modic MT, et al: Intravenous digital subtraction angiography application to cerebrovascular surgery. *Neurosurgery* 9:129–136, 1981.
14. Duff TA, Turski PA, Sackett JF et al: Evolving role of digital subtraction angiography in neurosurgical practice. *Neurosurgery* 11:430–438, 1982.
15. Seeger JF, Weinstein PR, Carmody RF, et al: Digital video subtraction angiography of the cervical and cerebral vasculature. *J Neurosurg* 56:173–179, 1982.
16. Carmody RD, Smith JRL, Seeger JF, et al: Intracranial applications of digital intravenous subtraction angiography. *Radiology* 144:529–534, 1982.
17. Enzmann DR, Brody WR, Riederer S, et al: Intracaranial intravenous digital subtraction angiography. *Neuroradiology* 23:241–251, 1982.
18. De Filipp G, Pinto RS, Lin JP, et al: Intravenous digital subtraction angiography in the investigation of intracranial disease. *Radiology* 148:129–136, 1983.
19. Forbes G, Earnest F, Kispert D, et al: Digital angiography: Introducing digital techniques to clinical cerebral angiography practice. *Mayo Clin Proc* 57:683–693, 1982.
20. DeLahitte MD, Marc-Vergnes JP, Rascol A, et al: Intravenous angiography of the extracranial cerebral arteries. *Radiology* 137:705–711, 1980.
21. Sheldon JJ, Janowitz W, Leborgne JM, et al: Intravenous DSA of extracranial carotid lesions: Comparison with other techniques and specimens. *AJR* 143:1289–1294, 1984.
22. Miller RW, Carmody RF, Seeger JS, et al: Digital subtraction angiography: Applications in otolaryngology—head and neck surgery. *Head Neck Surg* 5:280–292, 1983.
23. Kinney SE, Modic MT, Starnes D, et al: Digital subtraction angiography of lesions of the head and neck. *Laryngoscope* 92:557–561, 1982.
24. Campo RV, Reeser FH: Retinal telangiectasias secondary to bilateral carotid artery occlusion. *Arch Ophthalmol* 101:1211–1213, 1983.
25. Shah HG, Brown GC, Goldberg RE: Digital subtraction carotid angiography and retinal arterial obstruction. *Ophalmology* 92:68–72, 1985.
26. Lee BCP, Voorhies TM, Ehrlich ME, et al: Digital intravenous cerebral angiography in neonates. *AJNR* 5:281–286, 1984.
27. Wagner ML, Singleton EB, Egan ME: Digital subtraction angiography in children. *AJR* 140:127–133, 1983.
28. Faerber EN, Giska LAB, Swartz JD, et al: Digital subtraction angiography in pediatric cerebrovascular occlusive disease. *Radiology* 152:391–394, 1984.
29. Amundson GM, Wesenberg RL, Mueller DL, et al: Pediatric digital subtraction angiography. *Radiology* 153:649–654, 1984.
30. Capitanio MA, Faerber EN, Gainey MA, et al: Digital subtraction angiography and its application in children. *Pediatr Clin North Am* 32:1449–1460, 1985.
31. Mueller DL, Amundson GM, Wesenberg RL, et al: The application of IV digital subtraction angiography to cranial disease in children. *AJNR* 7:669–674, 1986.
32. Rosenblum J, Yousefzadeh DK, Ramilo JL: Skull radiography in infants: Potential hazards of the use of head clamps. *Radiology* 161:367–368, 1986.
33. Enzmann DR, Freimarck R: Head immobilization for digital subtraction angiography. *Radiology* 151:801, 1984.
34. Katzen BT: Peripheral, abdominal and interventional applications of DS. *Radiol Clin North Am* 23:227–241, 1985.
35. Thompson JR, Schneider S, Ashwal S, et al: The choice of sedation for computed tomography in children: a prospective evaluation. *Radiology* 143:475–479, 1982.
36. Davis PC, Hoffman JC Jr: Work in progress: Intraarterial digital subtraction angiography: Evaluation in 150 patients. *Radiology* 148:9–15, 1983.
37. Bunker SR, Cutaia FI, Fritz AL: Femoral intraarterial digital angiography: an outpatient procedure. *AJR* 141:593–596, 1983.
38. Flannigan BD, Gomes AS, Stambuk EL, et al: Intraarterial digital subtraction angiography: Comparison with conventional hepatic angiography. *Radiology* 148:17–21, 1983.
39. Miller FJ, Mineau DE, Koehler PR: Clinical intraarterial digital subtraction imaging. *Radiology* 148:273–278, 1983.

40. Weinstein MA, Pavlicek WA, Modk MT, et al: Intraarterial digital subtraction angiography of the head and neck. *Radiology* 147:717–724, 1983.
41. Brant-Zawadzki M, Gould R, Norman D, et al: Digital subtraction cerebral angiography of intraarterial injection: Comparison with conventional angiography. *AJR* 140:347–352, 1983.
42. Crummy AB, Stieghorst MF, Turski PA, et al: Digital subtraction angiography: Current status and use of intraarterial injection. *Radiology* 145:303–307, 1982.
43. Pelz DM, Fox AJ, Vinuela F: Techniques and risks of cerebral angiography. In Taveras M, Ferrucci JT (Eds): *Radiology, Diagnosis-Imaging-Intervention*. Philadelphia, J. B. Lippincott, 1986, pp. 1–14.
44. Franken EA Jr, Girod D, Sequera FW, et al: Femoral artery spasm in children: Catheter size is the principal cause. *AJR* 138:295–298, 1982.
45. Rubin DL, Burbank FH, Bradley BR, et al: An experimental evaluation of central vs. peripheral injection for intravenous digital subtraction angiography (IV-DSA). *Invest Radiol* 19:30–35, 1984.
46. Kadir S: Digital subtraction angiography (DSA). In: *Diagnostic Angiography*, Philadelphia, PA: W. B. Saunders & Co., 1986, pp. 103–123.
47. Rosen RJ, Miller DL, DeFilipp G: Mediastinal extravasation during digital angiography. *AJR* 140:389–390, 1983.
48. Modic MT, Weinstein MA, Pavlicek W, et al: Intravenous digital subtraction angiography: Peripheral vs. cerebral injection of contrast material. *Radiology* 147:711–715, 1983.
49. Smergel E: Digital subtraction angiography of the extremities. In Faerber EN (Ed): *Digital Subtraction Imaging in Infants and Children*. Mt. Kisco, NY: Futura Publishing Co., Inc. 1988, pp. .
50. Hayman LA, Hinck L: Central nervous system angiography: Contrast media. In Taveras M, Ferrucci JT (Eds): *Radiology, Diagnosis-Imaging-Intervention*. Philadelphia, PA: J. B. Lippincott, 1986, pp. 1–5.
51. Carmody RF, Seeger JF: Intracranial applications of digital subtraction angiography. *CRC Crit Rev Diagn Imaging* 23:1–40, 1984.
52. Modic MT, Weinstein MA, Chilcote WA, et al: Digital subtraction angiography of the intracranial vascular system: Comparative study in 55 patients. *AJR* 138:299–306, 1982.
53. Takahashi M, Hirota Y, Bussaka H, et al: Evaluation of prototype equipment for digital subtraction angiography in diagnosing intracranial lesions. *AJNR* 4:259–262, 1983.
54. Enzmann DR, Brody WR, Riederer S, Collins W, Pelc N: Intracranial intravenous digital subtraction angiography. *Neuroradiology* 23:241–251, 1982.
55. Pinto RS, Kricheff II, DeFilipp G, et al: Vasospasm secondary to ruptured aneurysm: Assessment by digital intravenous angiography. *AJNR* 4:283–285, 1983.
56. Butler P, Freer CEL, Jha AN, et al: Intravenous digital subtraction angiography in intracranial aneurysms. *Br J Radiol* 60:323–326, 1987.
57. Gardeur D: Tomodensitometrie intra-cranienne. Livre II—*Pathologie vasculaire*, vol 1. Paris: Ellipse, 1982.
58. Gardeur D, Seurot M, Fonda C, et al: Digital intravenous subtraction angiography of intracranial arteriovenous malformations. *Neuroradiology* 25:307–313, 1983.
59. Carmody RF, Smith JRL, Seeger JF, et al: Intracranial applications of digital intravenous subtraction angiography. *Radiology* 144:529–534, 1982.
60. Modic MT, Weinstein MA, Starnes DL, et al: Intravenous digital subtraction angiography of the intracranial veins and dural sinuses. *Radiology* 146:383–389, 1983.
61. Barnes BD, Brant-Zawadzki M, Mentzer W: Digital subtraction angiography in the diagnosis of superior sagittal sinus thrombosis. *Neurology* 33:508–510, 1983.
62. Schoenberg BS, Mellinger JF, Schoenberg DG: Cerebrovascular disease in infants and children: A study of incidence, clinical features and survival. *Neurology* 28:763–768, 1978.

63. Hilal SE, Solomon GE, Gold AP, et al: Primary cerebral arterial occlusive disease in children. Part I: Acute acquired hemiplegia. *Radiology* 99:71–86, 1971.
64. Richards D, Nulsen FE: Angiographic media and the sickling phenomenon. *Surg Forum* 22:403–404, 1971.
65. Korein J, Braunstein P, Kricheff II, et al: Radioisotope bolus technique as a test to detect circulatory deficit associated with cerebral death. *Circulation* 51:924–929, 1975.
66. Cranford RE, Smith HL: Some critical distinctions between brain death and the persistent vegetative state. *Soc Sci Med* 6:199–209, 1979.
67. Gomes AS, Hallinan JM: Intravenous digital subtraction angiography in the diagnosis of brain death. *AJNR* 4:21–24, 1983.
68. Vatne K, Nakstad P, Lundar T: Digital subtraction angiography (DSA) in the evaluation of brain death. *Neuroradiology* 27:155–157, 1985.
69. Neiman HL, Mintzer RA, Vogelzang RL: Digital subtraction angiography. In Neiman HL, Yao JST (Eds): Angiography of Vascular Disease. New York: Churchill-Livingstone, 1985, pp. 27–56.
70. Aaron JO, Taveras JM: The angiographic localization of supratentorial masses. In Taveras JM, Ferrucci JT (Eds): *Radiology, Diagnosis-Imaging-Intervention*. Philadelphia: JB Lippincott, 1986, pp. 1–9.
71. Pinto RS, Manuell M, Kricheff II: Complications of digital intravenous angiography: Experience in 2488 cervicocranial examinations. *AJR* 143:1295–1299, 1984.
72. Ball JB Jr, Lukin RR, Tomsick TA, et al: Complications of intravenous digital subtraction angiography. *Arch Neurol* 42:969–972, 1985.

Chapter 7

Renal Digital Subtraction Angiography

GRIGORY ROZENBLIT, THOMAS A. SOS, CALVIN D. NEITHAMER, JR., and KENNETH S. CRYSTAL

The diagnosis and treatment of renal macrovascular pathology is primarily, although not exclusively, determined by angiography. The methods of angiography include conventional techniques utilizing large format (14″ × 14″) film screen combinations, 105-mm 100 or spot film photofluorography, and, more recently, digital subtraction angiography (DSA). A safe and cost-effective application of DSA for renovascular disease necessitates a clear understanding of the advantages, disadvantages, and diagnostic capabilities of DSA.[1] These topics will be the subject of the following discussion.

Intravenous DSA

The major advantage of intravenous DSA (IVDSA) compared to conventional arterial angiography is its potentially safer catheterization approach. In addition, angiography performed by the intravenous route can often be done on an outpatient basis without having to admit the child to hospital. This important advantage, however, does not always compensate for the disadvantages of IVDSA which include loss of spatial resolution and the relatively high contrast load inherent in intravenous arteriography[2] (Fig. 1). In addition, patient motion (including respiratory), which is almost inevitable in small children, is particularly troublesome in IVDSA. Such motion results in misregistration artifacts which severely degrade digital renovascular images.[2–5] Because of these disadvantages, the use of IVDSA in the diagnosis of renovascular abnormalities in children is significantly limited (Fig. 2).

Intra-Arterial DSA

Intra-arterial DSA (IADSA) has a number of distinct advantages. Approximately six times less volume of contrast material is required when performing

Digital Subtraction Imaging in Infants and Children, edited by Eric N. Faerber. Mount Kisco, New York: Futura Publishing Company, Inc., © 1989.

IADSA as compared to arteriographic techniques and IVDSA.[4] In addition, IADSA images are less susceptible to degradation by motion than are IVDSA images. This is because imaging is performed immediately and more rapidly during contrast injection. Thus, good quality images can be acquired even in young or relatively uncooperative children. However, the information acquired by intra-aortic IADSA may also be insufficient for reaching a treatment decision since renal artery branches beyond the segmental ones may be poorly seen.[5,6] Therefore, when visualization of relatively small renal vessels is essential even selective IADSA cannot be used alone because of possible artifacts but may have to be followed by selective conventional angiography.

For the correct application of DSA, a basic understanding of renovascular pathology in the pediatric age group is essential. The pathologic conditions affecting the renal vessels are listed in Table 1. The indications for renal angiography are summarized in Table 2. Hypertension, which may be primary or secondary, is the most common indication for performing renal angiography in children.

Table 1. Renovascular Conditions Detected by Angiography

Arterial		Venous	Arteriovenous
Obstruction	Aneurysm	Congenital variants Thrombosis Extrinsic compression	Malformation Fistula
Fibromuscular dysplasia Arteritis Neurofibromatosis Dissection Embolism Thrombosis Atherosclerosis Post radiation Extrinsic compression Post traumatic & iatrogenic Transplant artery disease	Major Artery Idiopathic Fibromuscular dysplasia Arteritis Neurofibromatosis Small or Parenchymal Branch Polyarteritis nodosa		

Table 2. Indications for Renal Angiography

Diagnostic Evaluation of
- Hypertension
- Unexplained hematuria
- Unexplained impairment of renal function
- Suspected renovascular trauma
- Suspected polyarteritis nodosa
- Possible tumor

Posttherapeutic Evaluation
Preoperative Vascular Mapping

Renovascular Hypertension

Although all forms of hypertension may occur in pediatric patients, the hypertension in a child less than 10 years of age has a 50% to 80% probability of being secondary.[7–10] In contrast, hypertension in the adult is secondary in only 10% of cases. Renal vascular disease accounts for 10% to 75% of all cases of secondary hypertension.[7,11,12] Renovascular hypertension is thus relatively more common among hypertensive children than among hypertensive adults.

The most common etiology for renovascular hypertension is renal artery obstruction (stenosis or occlusion). Fibromuscular dysplasia constitutes 95% of the renal arterial obstructing lesions in the pediatric age group; the remaining 5% exhibit varying types of arteritis. Other causes of renovascular hypertension in children are uncommon.[9] In 25% to 64% of all renal arterial obstructive lesions, a segmental renal artery is involved. Of these, 25% to 43% involve a segmental branch only, with no abnormality of the main renal artery. In 25% to 40% of cases, renovascular disease is bilateral.[9,13,14]

When the peculiarities of renovascular hypertension in children as described above are considered, it is apparent that the algorithm of the angiographic work-up for this disorder in the pediatric age group will differ from that in adults. Since renovascular hypertension is a potentially curable condition, it must be excluded in every case of renin-mediated hypertension in children and adolescents. Therefore, renal vein renin (RVR) sampling will be required prior to performing angiography in order to determine the site of renin hypersecretion. When RVR sampling is performed correctly, it is very sensitive and specific.[15] In our series of 11 pediatric patients with proven renovascular hypertension, RVR sampling showed true positive results in 10 children and equivocal values in 1 child.

As noted above, fibromuscular dysplasia is a common cause of renovascular hypertension in the pediatric age group. This disorder often involves the small intrarenal branches, and when fibromuscular dysplasia occurs in the main renal artery it may present as a subtle web or beading. Given the inherent low spatial resolution of DSA, such lesions may not be visualized utilizing this technique. Therefore, selective conventional film screen angiographic techniques and small focal spot magnification views may be required (Fig. 3) even. The use of these meticulous techniques, however, do not always clearly demonstrate the lesion which may be obscured by superimposition of "beads" as well as other arterial branches.[16] In our experience, the careful reevaluation of the angiogram and multiple selective arteriographic magnification views prompted by the positive results of RVR sampling with a captopril challenge test led to the demonstration of a previously missed lesion (Fig. 4).

IADSA, however, can be used in conjunction with other angiographic techniques resulting in a decrease in the total contrast load to the patient. For instance, digital aortography performed prior to selective renal angiography considerably reduces the amount of injected contrast, while diminishing discomfort to the patient. At the same time, the number and distribution of the renal arteries and lesions involving large renal vessels and aorta such as coarctation, hypoplasia, and arteritis can be demonstrated (Fig. 5). This approach is applicable to other renal arterial lesions that cause hypertension in children (Table 1).

After the diagnosis has been established and the morphology of the lesion has been demonstrated by conventional angiography, DSA can be a valuable adjunct to renal angioplasty.[17,18] Technically adequate online images can be obtained prior to and following balloon inflations employing a small image intensifier field size for better spatial resolution. Postdilation DSA can be safely performed by injecting through the balloon catheter, significantly decreasing the time required for angioplasty (Fig. 5). In addition, with some DSA systems, a preceding subtaction angiogram can be used as a mask for subsequent dynamic subtraction "road map" fluoroscopy, which allows for precise, fast, and convenient balloon positioning during angioplasty.[4,6]

Renovascular Disease with Hypertension

In addition to hypertension, renal vascular abnormalities may present with a variety of other manifestations. Unexplained hematuria or impaired renal function, suspected renovascular trauma, or polyarteritis nodosa may prompt angiography to identify possibly curable lesions.

The diagnostic angiographic approach will depend on the pathology suspected of being present. If abnormalities of the major renal vessels are suspected, such as posttraumatic renal artery occlusion or aortic occlusion, IADSA may be sufficient for diagnosis (Fig. 6). Although IVDSA may demonstrate interruption of vascular blood flow under favorable circumstances, it is a less reliable angiographic method. Important information which could be critical for treatment decisions, such as occlusion of an accessory renal artery or distal reconstitution of a proximally occluded artery, may be missed utilizing IVDSA.[3]

If the demonstration of fine vascular detail is essential for diagnosis and/or management, conventional angiography often with small focal spot magnification technique is indicated. As noted above, however, IADSA may be used advantageously in conjunction with conventional angiographic techniques.

When the demonstration of a major renal vein is necessary, as in thrombosis or extrinsic compression, digital venography can be performed. The contrast material is administered directly in the area of interest, the renal vein, and is analogous to IADSA in both spatial resolution and contrast load.

Post-Therapeutic Evaluation

Digital angiography can be employed for follow-up after radiologic renovascular interventional procedures (angioplasty, thrombolysis, or embolization), vascular reconstructive surgery, or renal transplant.[19–22] DSA can be performed either as a baseline study or following recurrence of symptoms. The precise location of the lesion, its morphologic characteristics and anatomy are already known and comparison with a previous angiogram is usually possible. These factors may make IVDSA quite applicable for posttherapeutic evaluation. Because the angiographic appearance of the area of interest is already known, it is possible to utilize the smallest possible image intensifier field size with a resultant increase in spatial resolution. The precise understanding of the three-dimensional anatomy of the area of interest permits imaging in an optimal projection. This allows for improved visualization of anatomic detail and at the same time reduces the number of injections and overall contrast load to the patient. Knowledge of the morphologic characteristics of the lesion and the availability of a previous study for comparison facilitate "pattern recognition" and assessment of interval changes by the radiologist and decrease the possibility of misinterpretation.

IVDSA is very sensitive and quite specific for follow-up after renovascular intervention and renal transplant surgery.[23] In those few instances when the results of IVDSA are indeterminate or when better visualization of fine detail is required, it may be followed by IADSA. On the other hand, the main advantages of IVDSA, namely its safer catheterization approach and the ability to perform the study on an outpatient basis, become very important for post-therapeutic evaluation. Therefore, IVDSA is often the procedure of choice for postinterventional follow-up, decreasing the risk, cost, and inconvenience of angiography.

An understanding of the capabilities and limitations of DSA will result in the appropriate, safe, beneficial, and cost-effective application for renal angiography in the pediatric age group.

Preoperative Vascular Mapping

Angiography for preoperative vascular mapping is usually requested in two clinical situations: evaluation of a potential renal donor (older teenagers or adults) and prior to partial nephrectomy.

Angiography in a potential renal donor may be performed by means of IVDSA. This method, however, has an accuracy of only 86% and an accessory renal artery which may be small or out of the field of view could be easily missed[11] (Fig. 7). Therefore, in our institution, potential renal donors are evaluated by conventional aortography and, if indicated, by selective arteriography. It is conceivable, however, that the application of a larger size image intensifier field (14.5 in) would allow for the use of IADSA instead of conventional aortography in the evaluation of a potential renal donor.

Vascular mapping prior to partial nephrectomy requires the demonstration of three-dimensional vascular anatomy. To achieve this, intra-arterial multiprojectional angiography is essential. This can be performed using either digital or conventional angiographic techniques. At times, superselective injections are necessary in order to achieve accurate vascular mapping. In general, IADSA is the preferred technique since the amount of contrast material used for the study can be significantly reduced when utilizing this imaging modality. IVDSA plays no role in vascular mapping prior to partial nephrectomy.

Conclusion

DSA is an important radiologic method for the diagnosis, interventional treatment, and follow-up of renal vascular abnormalities in the pediatric age group.

IVDSA has limited applications in renal angiography, especially in young children. It can be useful in the older age groups, however, for posttherapeutic evaluation.

IADSA is an essential part of contemporary general angiography in children. It is the preferred imaging technique for the diagnosis of major renal artery lesions such as traumatic occlusion. IADSA is a valuable adjunct to conventional angiographic techniques. At times IADSA may be used instead of conventional angiography, significantly reducing the overall contrast load to the patient. Lastly, IADSA can be a very useful technique for online imaging during renal vascular interventional procedures.

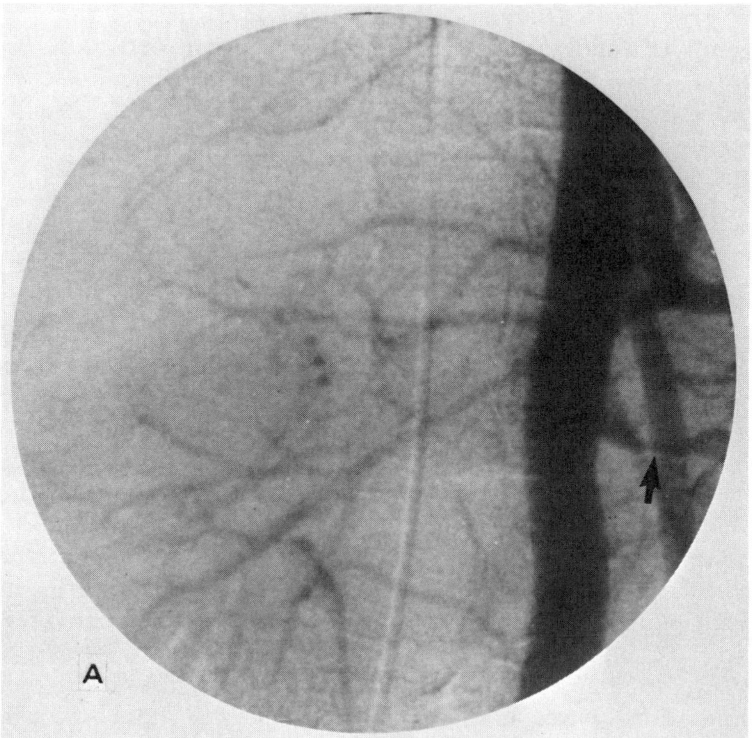

FIGURE 1. Seventeen-year-old female with recently discovered hypertension (201/120 mmHg). Bilateral renal artery stenosis due to fibromuscular dysplasia. **A**: *The IVDSA shows left renal artery stenosis (arrow) but fails to demonstrate the anatomy and severity of the lesion on the right side.* **B**: *The aortogram reveals high degree stenosis (arrow) with collaterals (curved arrows) filling the lower pole branch (open arrow) on the right side. Left main renal artery stenosis is also well visualized.* **C**: *The postangioplasty aortogram demonstrates no evidence of residual hemodynamically significant lesions in the main renal arteries on either side. There is mild segmental artery stenosis on the left. (arrow).*

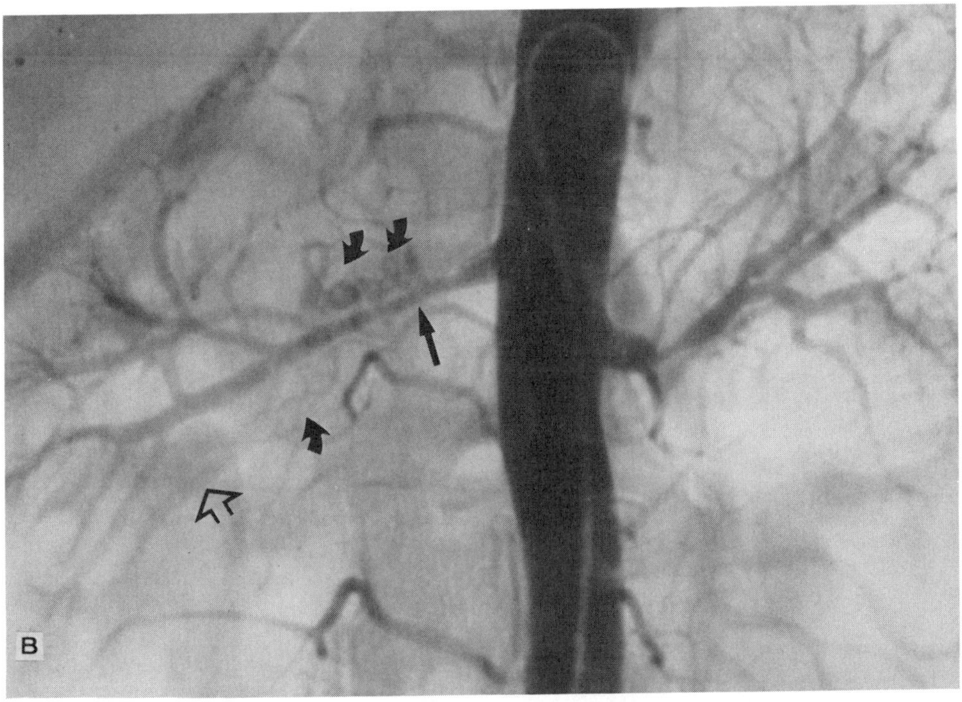

FIGURE 1B.

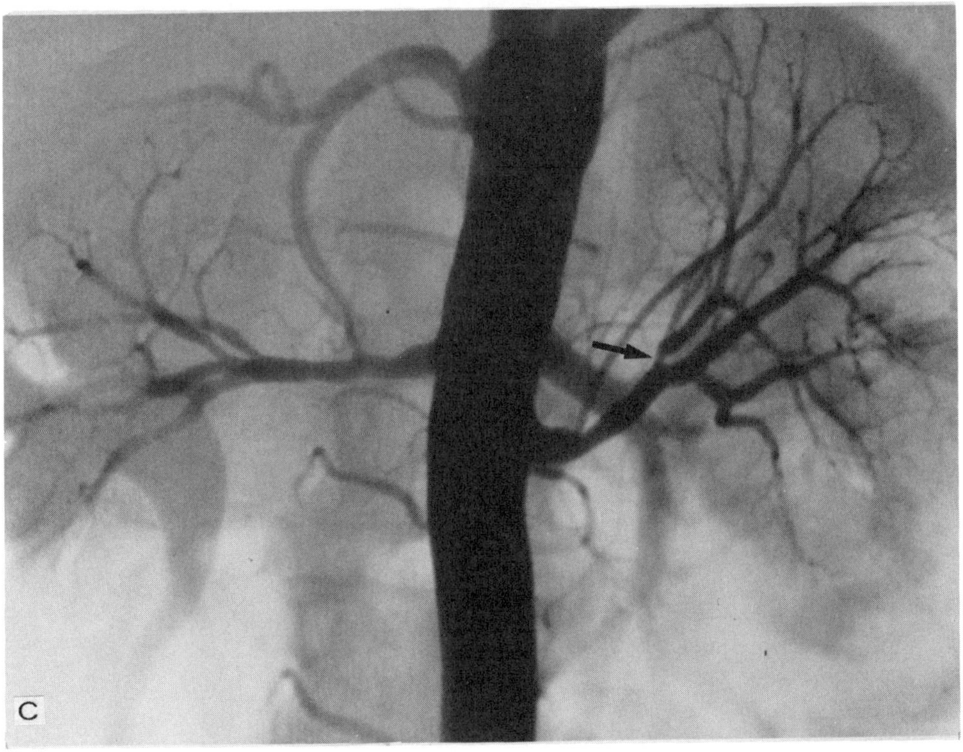

FIGURE 1C.

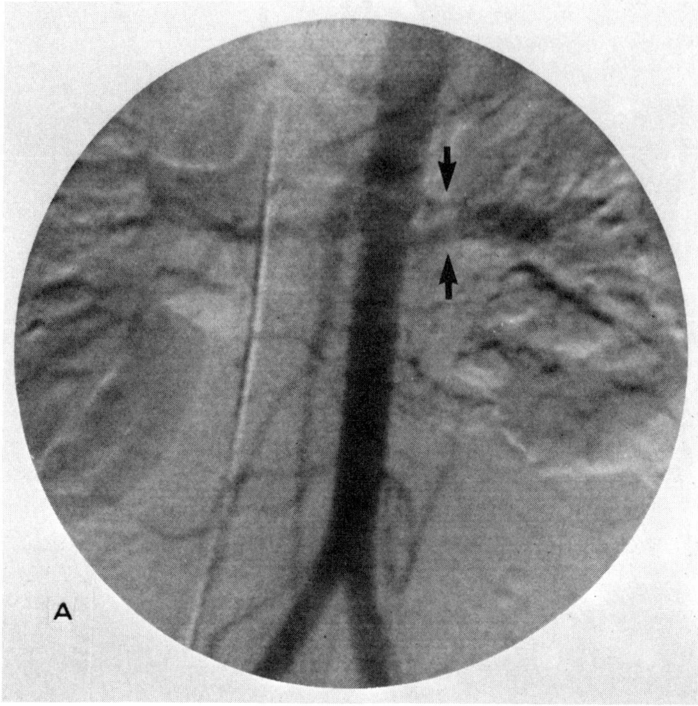

A

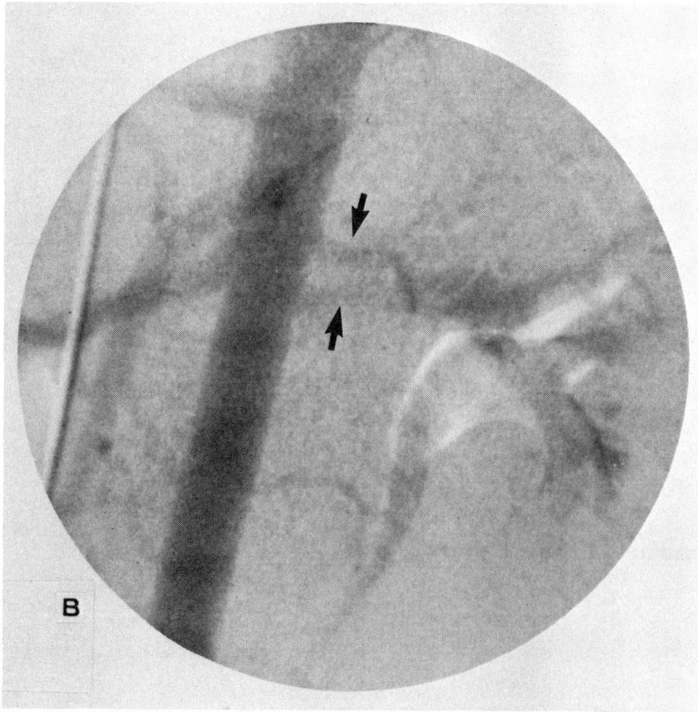

B

FIGURE 2. Fifteen-year-old female with three-year history of hypertension. **A**: *Frontal and* **B**: *Left anterior oblique IVDSA demonstrate two left renal arteries (arrows); the inferior one has aneurysmal dilatation. However, definitive evaluation of these lesions is not possible despite several injections.* **C**: *The aortogram in frontal view defines the lesions better than IVDSA and confirms the presence of two left renal arteries. Note that even the aortogram does not allow reliable estimation of the degree of stenosis or visualization of the anatomical details.* **D**: *Selective left lower renal arteriogram demonstrates severe main artery stenosis (arrow) with collaterals (curved arrows) and a poststenotic aneurysm (open arrow). The segmental renal arteries (arrowheads) arise from the aneurysm.*

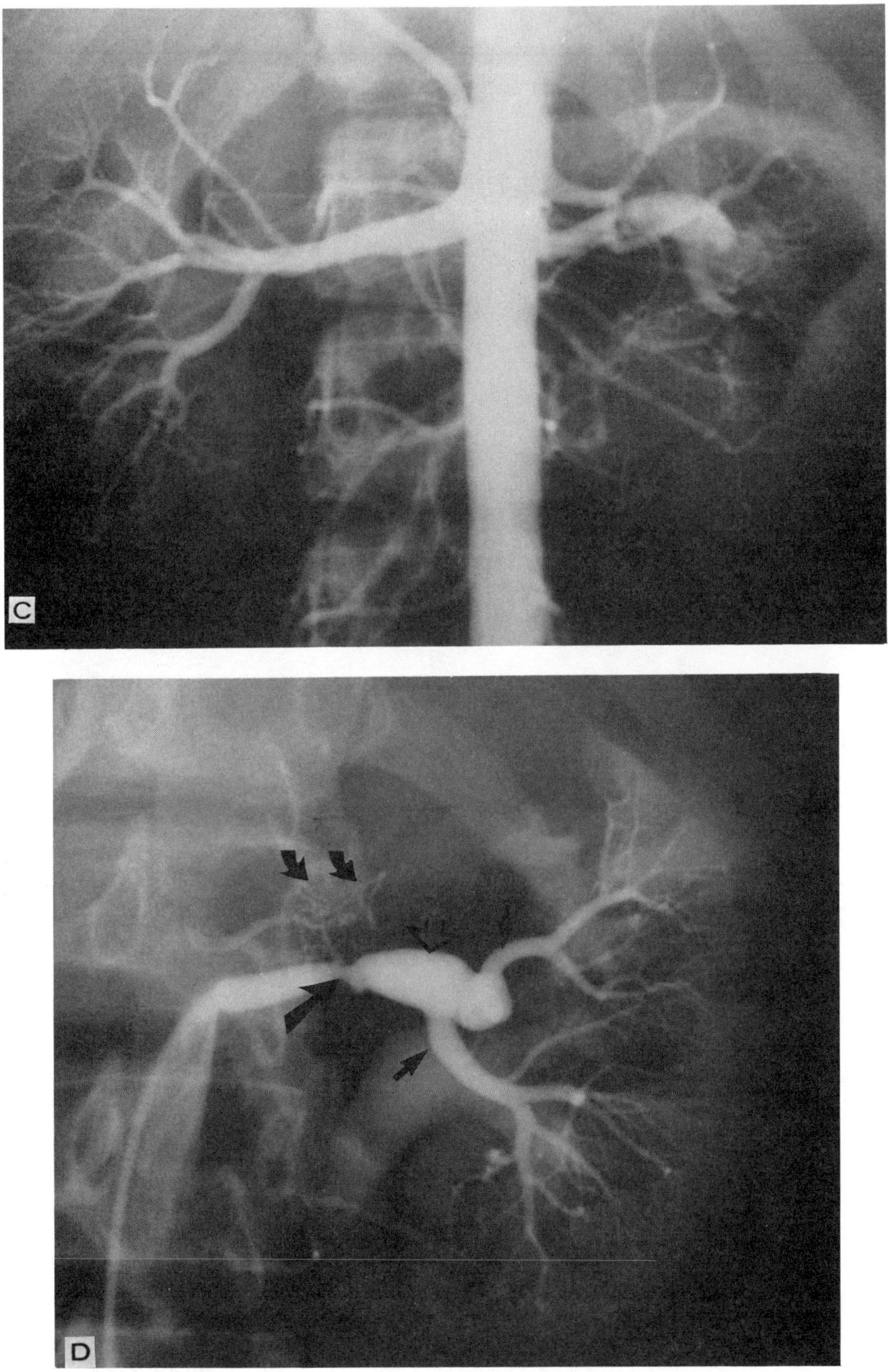

FIGURES 2C, D.

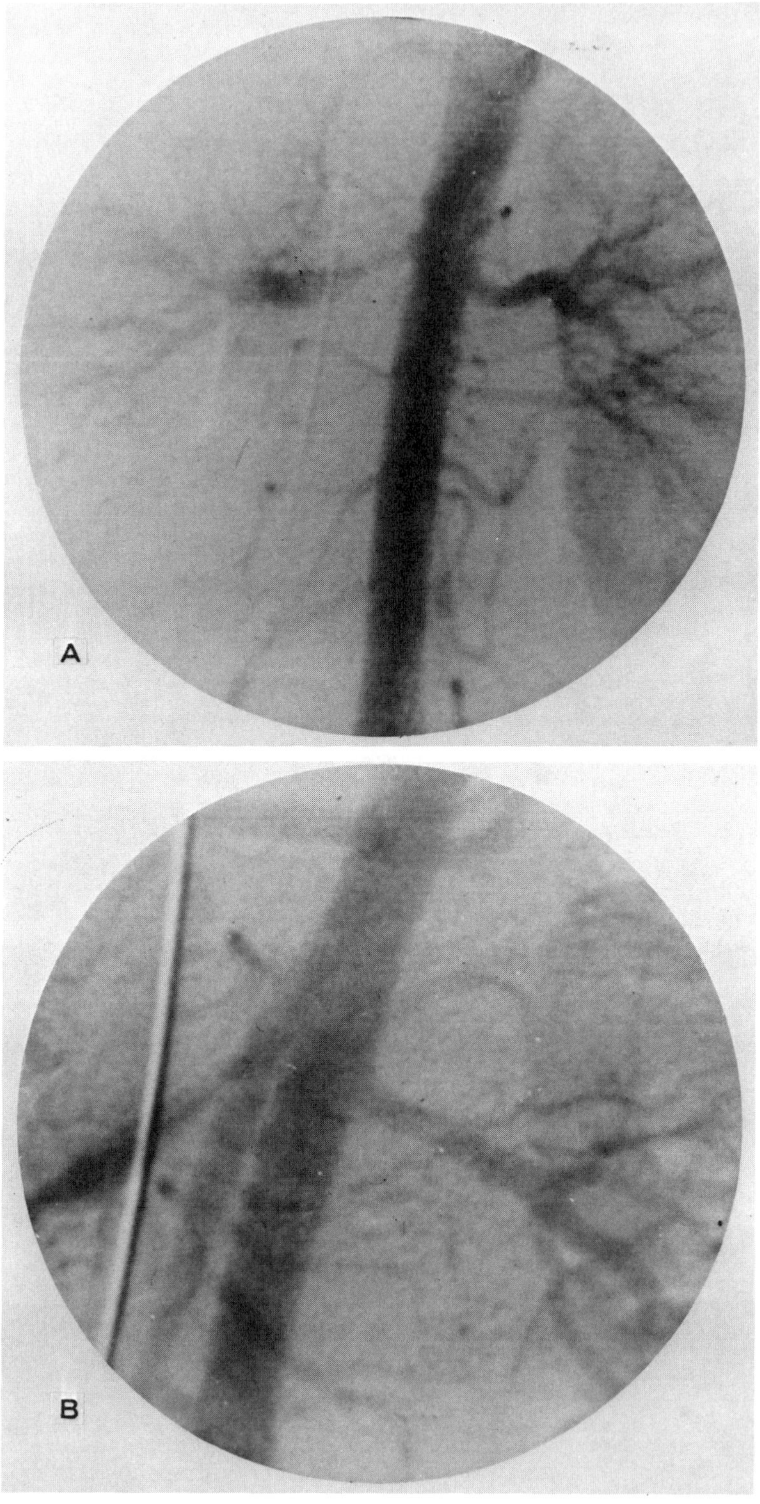

Figures 3A, B.

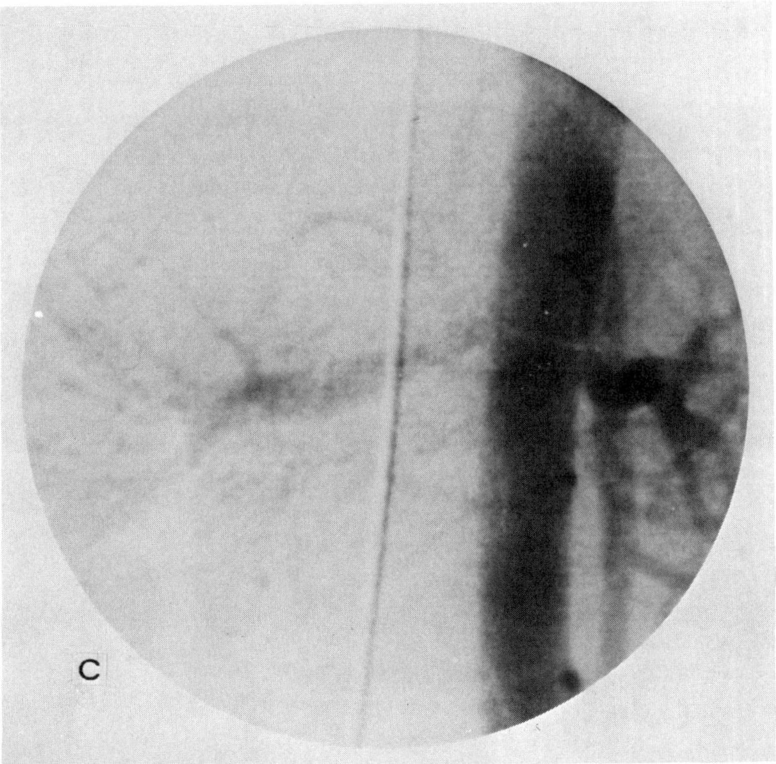

FIGURE 3. *Fifteen-year-old female with two-year history of hypertension with selective renins lateralizing to the right.* **A**, **B**, **C**: *AP and bilateral oblique IVDSA reveal a right main renal artery stenosis with poststenotic dilatation.* **D**: *The aortogram confirms the presence of right renal artery stenosis (arrow) with poststenotic dilatation (curved arrow) and collateral circulation (arrowheads). In addition, it demonstrates some irregularity of the main left renal artery (open arrow). This could be attributed to overlapping of different segments of the artery in frontal projection.* **E**: *The selective arteriogram clearly demonstrates the weblike lesion (arrowhead).*

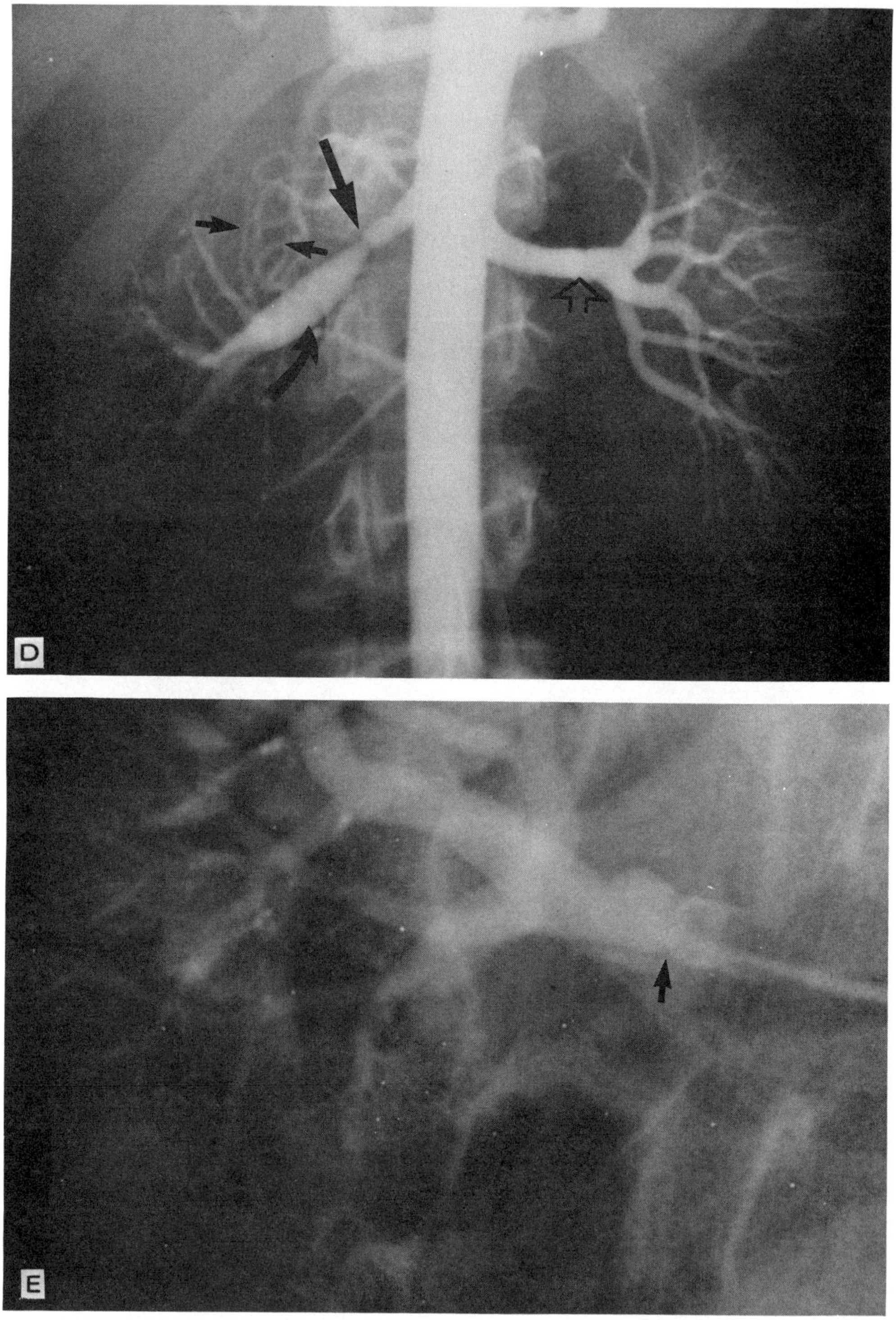

Figures 3D, E.

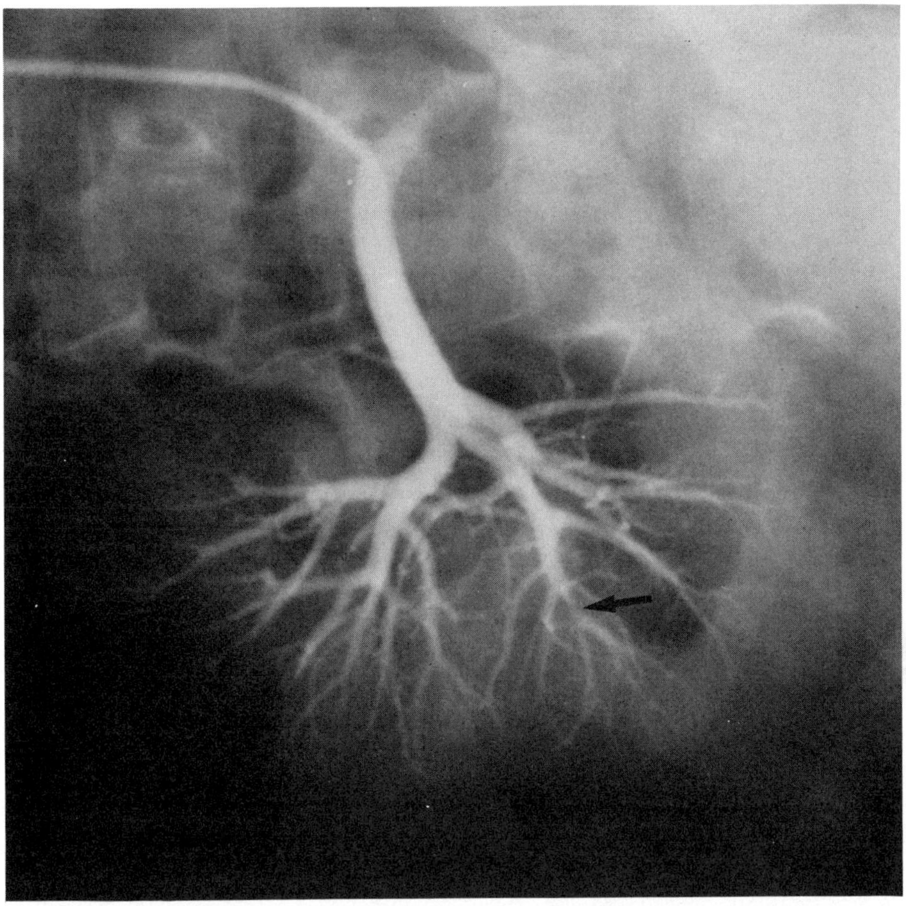

FIGURE 4. *Four-year-old female with a seven-week history of hypertension 130/100 mmHg, high peripheral renin, and positive captopril challenge test. A severe branch lesion (arrow) is very well visualized on this selective angiogram with small focal spot magnification. Such a lesion could be easily missed on an aortogram, or "masked" by superimposed branches if the images were acquired in one view only. IV or IADSA would both probably miss this very important lesion.*

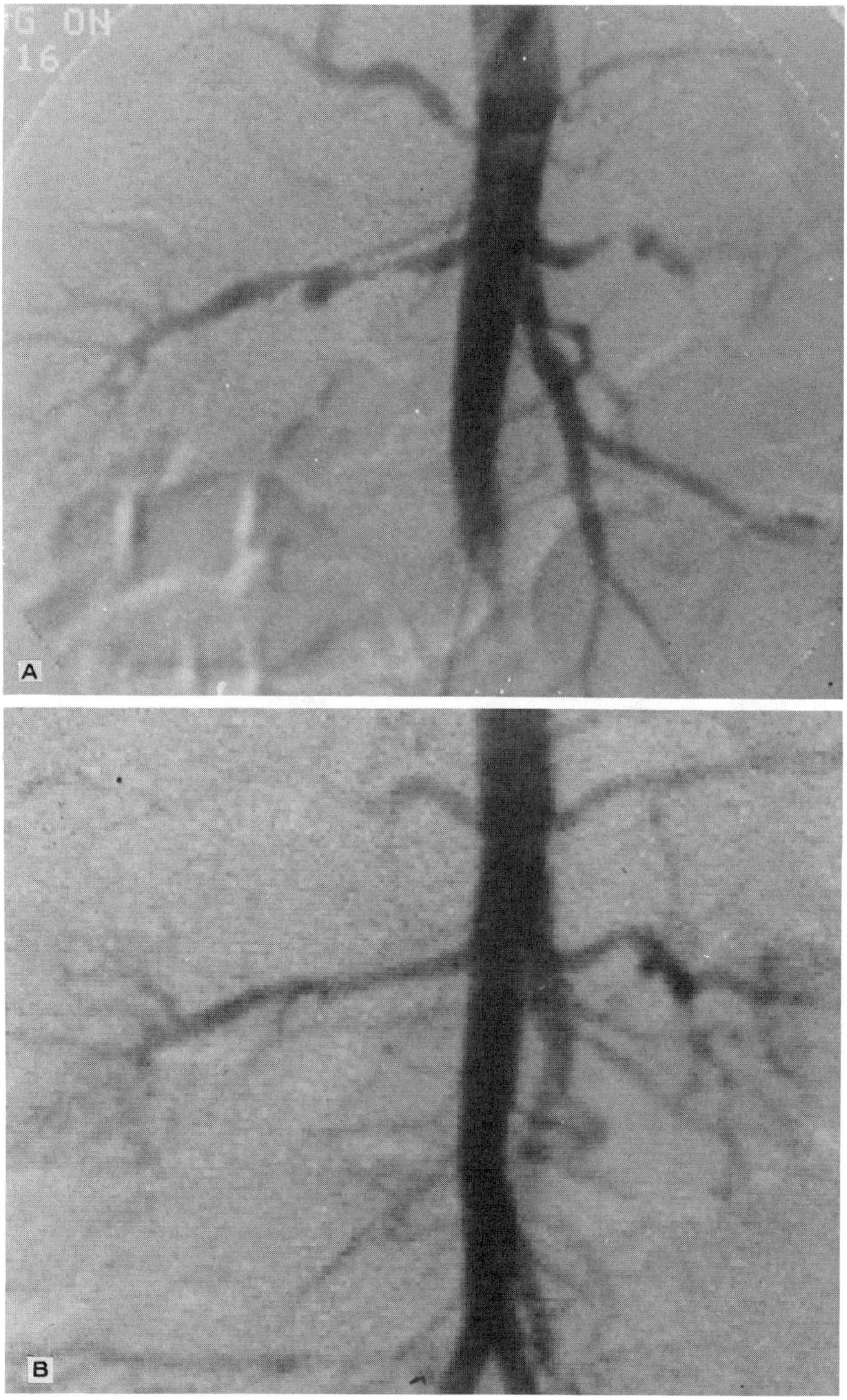

FIGURE 5. *Ten-month-old male with hypertension and history of intracerebral hemorrhage.* **A**: *The IADSA performed prior to angioplasty demonstrates single renal arteries with bilateral renal artery stenosis as well as an aneurysm on the right. Note also common hepatic artery stenosis.* **B**: *Postangioplasty. The IADSA demonstrates successful "cosmetic" dilation bilaterally.*

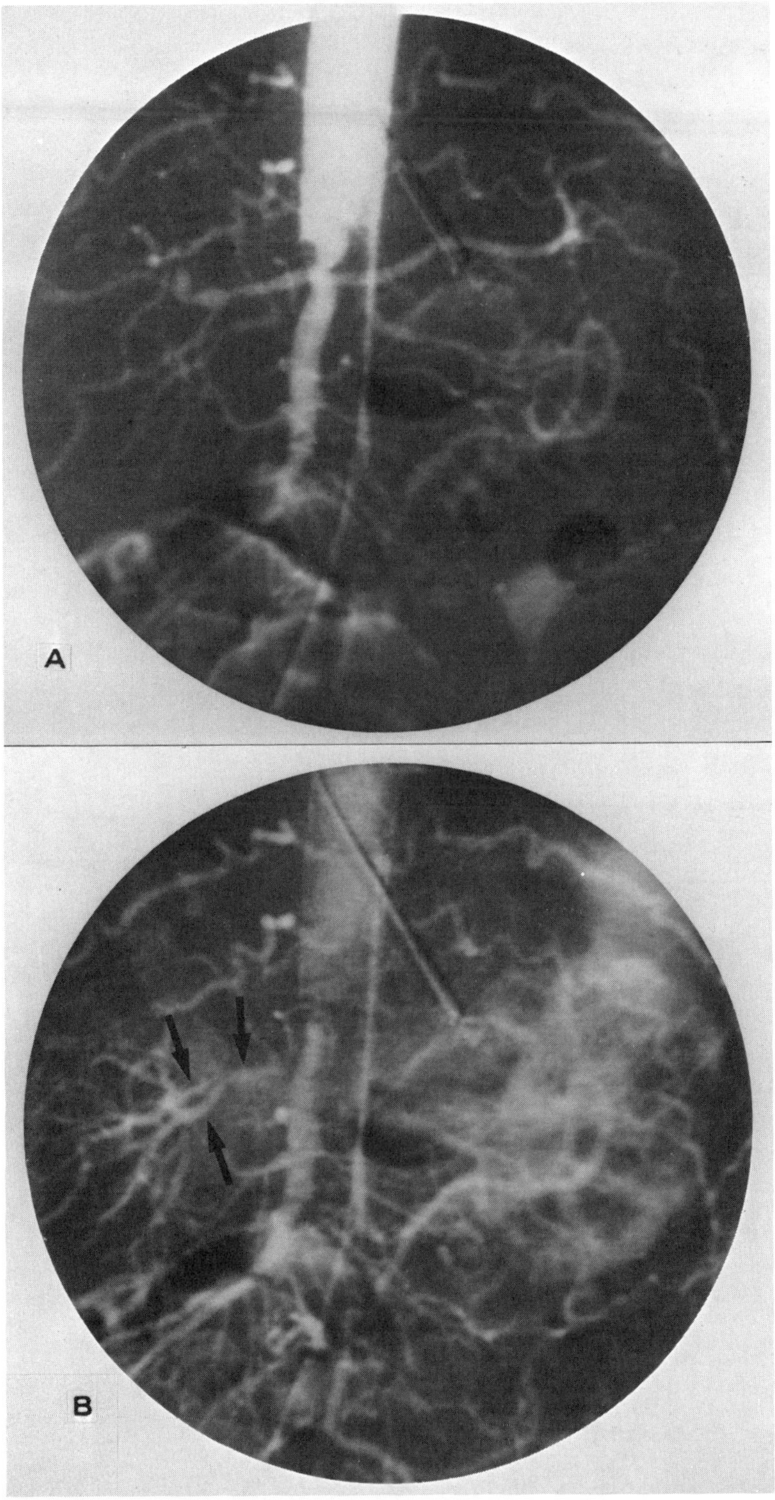

FIGURE 6. Ten-day-old male with suggested aortic thrombosis due to umbilical artery catheter. IADSA demonstrates aortic thrombosis. Both renal arteries are occluded at their origins with distal reconstitution of the right renal artery (arrows).

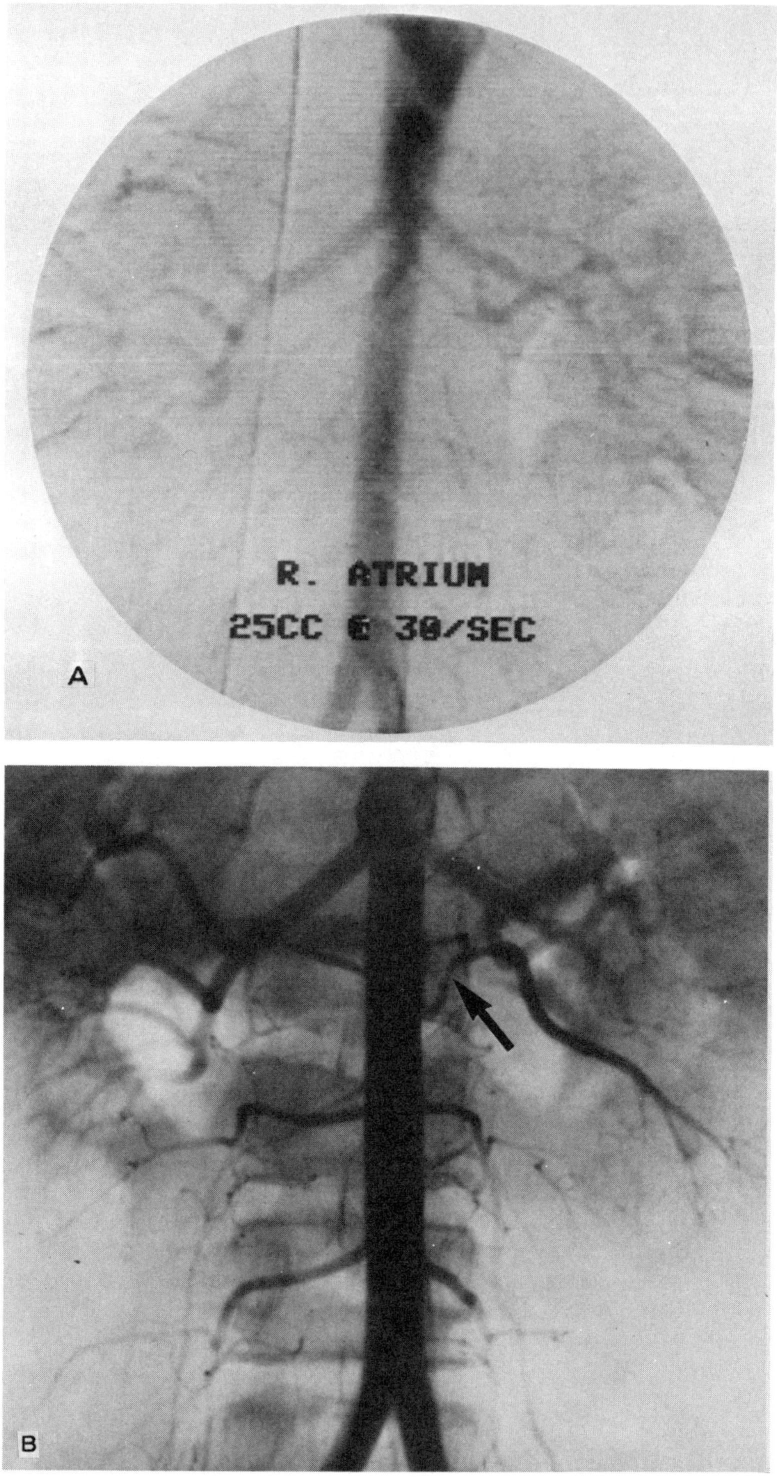

FIGURE 7. Fourteen-year-old female with blood pressure 160/100 mmHg. **A**: *The IVDSA failed to demonstrate the second renal artery on the left side.* **B**: *Aortogram reveals the accessory lower renal artery with severe stenosis on the left side (arrow).*

References

1. Buonocore E, Meaney TF, Borkowski GP, et al: Digital subtraction angiography of the abdominal aorta and renal arteries: Comparison with conventional aortography. *Radiology* 139:281–286, 1981.
2. Saddekni S, Sos TA, Srur M, et al: Contrast administration and techniques of digital subtraction angiography performance. *Radiol Clin North Am* 23:275–291, 1985.
3. Hillman BJ: Digital radiology of the kidney. *Radiol Clin North Am* 23:211–226, 1985.
4. Amundson GM, Wesenberg RL, Mueller DL, et al: Pediatric digital subtraction angiography. *Radiology* 153:649–654, 1984.
5. Capitanio MA, Faerber EN, Gainey MA, et al: Digital subtraction angiography and its application in children. *Pediatr Clin North Am* 32:1449–1460, 1985.
6. Foley WD, Milde MW: Intra-arterial digital subtraction angiography. *Radiol Clin North Am* 23:293–319, 1985.
7. Olson DI, Lieberman E: Renal hypertension in children. *Pediatr Clin North Am* 23:795–805, 1976.
8. Stanley P, Gyepes MT, Olson DL, et al: Renovascular hypertension in children and adolescents. *Radiology* 129:123–131, 1978.
9. Stanley JC: Renal vascular disease and renovascular hypertension in children. *Urol Clin North Am* 11:451–463, 1984.
10. Gomes AS, Pais SO, Barbaric ZL: Digital subtraction angiography in the evaluation of hypertension. *AJR* 140:779–783, 1983.
11. Lawson JD, Boerth R, Foster JH, et al: Diagnosis and management of renovascular hypertension in children. *Arch Surg* 112:1307–1316, 1977.
12. Foster JH, Pettinger WA, Oates JA, et al: Malignant hypertension secondary to renal artery stenosis in children. *Ann Surg* 164:700–713, 1966.
13. Clayman MD, Bookstein JJ: The role of renal arteriography in pediatric hypertension. *Radiology* 108:107–110, 1973.
14. Campbell DR, Mason WF, Flemming BK, et al: Digital subtraction arteriography in the diagnosis of renovascular hypertension. *J Can Assoc Radiol* 34:261–263, 1983.
15. Wenting GJ, Tan-Tjiong HL, Derkz FHM: Split renal function after captoprill in unilateral renal artery stenosis. *Br Med J* 288:886–889, 1984.
16. Busch HP, Strass LF, Hoevels J, et al: Fibromuscular dysplasia, a pitfall in intravenous digital subtraction angiography. *Eur J Radiol* 4:42–43, 1984.
17. Campbell DR, Mason QF, Flemming BK: Digital subtraction arteriography (DSA) in reevaluation of angioplasties. *J Can Assoc Radiol* 34:258–259, 1983.
18. Schwarten DE: Percutaneous transluminal angioplasty of the renal arteries: Intravenous digital subtraction angiography for follow-up. *Radiology* 150:369–373, 1984.
19. Jackson B, Dugdale L: Renal artery digital subtraction angiography: Outpatient investigation for renovascular hypertension. *Med J Aust* 142:18–21, 1985.
20. Novick AC, Buonocore E, Meaney TF: Digital subtraction angiography for postoperative evaluation of renal arterial reconstruction. *J Urol* 127:14–17, 1982.
21. Flechner SM, Novick AC, Meaney TF, et al: Simultaneous structural and functional imaging of the transplant kidney using digital subtraction angiography. *J Urol* 129:248–252, 1983.
22. Rath M, Castro L, Schuler M, et al: Digital subtraction angiography in the diagnosis of arterial complications after renal transplantation. *Eur J Radiol* 4:34–37, 1984.
23. Hillman BJ: Digital imaging of the kidney. *Radiol Clin North Am* 22:341–364, 1984.

Chapter 8

Digital Subtraction Angiography of the Extremities

ELEANOR MALONEY SMERGEL

Introduction

The applicability of digital subtraction angiography (DSA) to the extremities was reported in adults, with emphasis on peripheral vascular disease.[1–6] With time, applications to the extremities in children have been reported.[7] Although it has not proved to be completely ideal as an examination tool because of the limitation of spatial resolution and small field of view, DSA has been shown to be useful in evaluation of the extremities. In many cases, the limitations are offset by decreased risk to the patient and ease of performance of the study when compared to conventional angiography.

Technique

Careful selection of patients, adequate sedation, and attention to technical detail are important to ensure optimal results. The choice of intra-arterial versus intravenous injection will depend on the information required, on the status of the patient, and on the need to combine DSA with conventional or interventional procedures.[8]

Before the examination, history of allergies or previous contrast reaction is ascertained, as well as any history of renal disease, diabetes, or bleeding diatheses. If the study is to be by intravenous injection, no preliminary laboratory tests are routinely required. For an intra-arterial study, PT, PTT, and hemoglobin are checked beforehand. For elective studies, the patient is allowed nothing by mouth for three to four hours prior to the examination.

Sedation may not be necessary in the newborn infant. Older infants may be given chloral hydrate (80–100 mg/kg PO),[9] and children are usually sedated

Digital Subtraction Imaging in Infants and Children, edited by Eric N. Faerber. Mount Kisco, New York: Futura Publishing Company, Inc., © 1989.

with a cocktail containing Demerol (meperidine hydrochloride), 25 mg/mL, Phenergan (promethazine hydrochloride), 6.25 mg/mL, and Thorazine (chlorpromazine), 6.25 mg/mL. This is given intramuscularly in a dose of 0.1 ml/kg up to a maximum dose of 2 mL.[10] If the patient is refractory to sedation, small doses of intravenous Valium (diazepam) can be added. General anesthesia is almost never necessary, although there may be an occasional patient who is very uncooperative and refractory to the usual sedative.

If an intravenous study is to be performed, a central injection is preferable to a peripheral injection,[11–14] especially to visualize small vascular detail,[15] although some have argued otherwise.[16] A straight catheter with sideholes is used, as its insertion is less painful and less traumatic than a pigtail catheter.[17] It may be placed in the inferior vena cava via the femoral vein or in the superior vena cava via antecubital puncture of the basilic or cephalic vein. In a child, the basilic vein often narrows in the axilla, and the cephalic vein may make an acute angle with the axillary vein and may narrow at this site[18]; therefore, the antecubital route for central injection may be more difficult than in the adult.[17]

Opacification of vessels with an intravenous injection is proportional to the volume and concentration of contrast.[19] The contrast material for venous injection is generally 76% iodinated contrast medium, although good results can be obtained with as low as 45% concentration. The injection volume is determined by the weight of the child; approximately 0.66 mL/kg is used. Flow rate is adjusted to deliver the volume in 1 sec or less for central injection. Intra-arterial studies require only small volumes of contrast and, therefore, small catheters may be used.[11] For arterial injection, 15% to 43% concentration may be used.[20,21] The total dose of 76% iodinated contrast is kept below 4 mL/kg; use of more dilute contrast allows proportionately more total volume to be administered, allowing leeway for additional injections.

Imaging is performed at 3 frames/sec with an appropriate time interval between injection and the first image. Intervals of 2 to 6 sec between the injection and imaging are appropriate following intravenous injection, with the delay time depending on the heart rate, site of injection, and area of interest. DSA of the distal aspects of the extremities may necessitate delay times of up to 6 sec.

Vascular lesions of the extremities in children are usually localized, and since children are small, it is usually possible to fit the entire region of interest in one field. If both legs are of interest, crossing the legs at the ankles will bring the vessels closer together and allow more to be included in a single frame.[22] If the lesion happens to be large, multiple injections may be required in order to image over adjacent areas. If the extremity does not fill the field of view, a uniform exposure over the entire field can be obtained by placing bolus bags (water-filled bags) adjacent to the extremity. This is important because overexposure at the edges of the field of view severely degrades the image.

Unsuccessful studies may be caused by the following: contrast extravasation, unsuccessful vein cannulation, patient motion, computer malfunction, insufficient bolus, and poor exposure parameters.[17,23] Contrast extravasation and unsuccessful vein cannulation are more likely to occur when using peripheral rather than central sites for injection. In a large adult series, incidence of extravasation in the arm was 5.2% and in the mediastinum 0.13%.[24]

Advantages

Intravenous DSA (IVDSA) allows a study to be performed without the risks associated with arterial injection, such as thrombosis, embolization, false aneurysm, spasm, and hematoma. In addition, the IVDSA can be performed on outpatients, greatly lowering the cost of examination and making the procedure more readily acceptable to patients and their families.

When an arterial approach is indicated, intra-arterial digital subtraction angiography (IADSA) affords some distinct advantages over conventional angiographic techniques. The arteries of very young children are more prone to spasm than those of adults. However, smaller catheters may be used for IADSA, thus lowering the risk of catheter-related injury.[25] IADSA also reduces the need for selective catheterization of vessels.[26] In addition, the amount of contrast used for IADSA is much less than for IVDSA or conventional angiography. The latter is of importance in young children since the volume of contrast medium that can be used may be a limiting factor in achieving a complete study.

The pain that is usually experienced by the patient during conventional angiography when injections of contrast medium are made into vessels of the extremities is avoided when IVDSA and IADSA are performed. The low concentration of contrast medium used for arterial injections does not cause the intense pain associated with the intra-arterial injection of undiluted contrast medium needed for conventional studies.[8,20] This factor aids in limiting motion artifact and thus reduces the chance of motion artifacts during digital subtraction imaging.

In addition, DSA is an effective complementary tool for use during conventional angiographic studies. Real-time display of the image and immediate replay of the injection shorten the procedure time and facilitate interventional studies. Test injections can be recorded and displayed for immediate analysis of anatomy. When subtracted from real-time fluoroscopy, the test injection also allows "road mapping" of vessels to guide selective catheterization.[27] In addition, the superior contrast resolution of IA- and IVDSA provides better visualization of tumor stains and draining veins.

The overall radiation dose to the patient during a DSA examination is less than the dose during conventional angiography. Although the radiation dose to the patient during digital imaging is comparable, significantly less fluoroscopic time is used with DSA, thus reducing the total radiation dose.[7]

The cost of DSA is also significantly less, mainly due to the fact that much less film is used than for conventional studies.[26] Since vessels are not selectively catheterized and immediate review of injection is possible, the examination time is reduced when DSA is utilized.

Limitations

When compared with conventional angiography, both IV- and IADSA suffer from poorer spatial resolution. The resolution of DSA is approximately 2 line pairs/mm, compared with 6 line pairs/mm.[12] The fine vasculature is therefore unsharp on a DSA study.

Although intensifiers up to 16 inches in diameter are being used for peripheral vasculature,[28] the small field size limits the portion of the anatomy that can be recorded at one time. Vessel overlap, which can limit DSA in certain regions of the body, is not usually a problem in the extremities.

Optimal DSA results are seriously impaired by any motion of the patient, and since children are often unable to cooperate, they usually need to be sedated. Cardiac and renal disease also impair the quality of IVDSA, but these problems are encountered much less frequently in children than in adults.

Applications

Trauma

As in the adult, traumatic vascular injuries in children often require immediate surgical or radiologic intervention in order to preserve total function of the extremity. Accepted indications for angiography following trauma to the extremities include: expanding hematoma, bruit, dimished pulse, neurologic deficit, or proximity of trauma to the path of a vessel.[29–32] Penetrating or blunt injuries can lead to transection of a vessel, pseudoaneurysm, arteriovenous fistula, or intramural hematoma or thrombosis.[33] Until recently, conventional angiography has been the means to define the nature and extent of vascular injury precisely.[34] DSA is now also available to evaluate the patient with suspected vascular injury to the extremities.[23,35] (Figs. 1–3). IV- or IADSA can be used and aneurysms, false aneurysms, and arteriovenous fistulas are readily seen.[36] IVDSA can show vascular lacerations, transection, arteriovenous fistulae, and thrombosis as sensitively as conventional angiography.[37] DSA, however, may miss small intimal flaps. Intimal tears are usually related to stretching of the vessel such as may be caused by blunt injury or injury by a penetrating object at high velocity; therefore, caution should be used in evaluating these injuries with DSA. Other forms of trauma such as thermal or electrical burn may damage vessels, generally resulting in occlusion. In such cases, DSA can aid in planning skin graft surgery by delineating vascular supply (Fig. 4).

Many vascular injuries in children are iatrogenic in origin,[38] and DSA has been used to study these lesions[39] (Fig. 5). Either vascular insufficiency due to occlusion or pseudoaneurysm can develop in infants after catheterization of the femoral or umbilical artery (Fig. 6). Absence of distal pulses or a cold, pale, or mottled limb indicates vascular compromise. IVDSA distinguishes between spasm and thrombosis, locates the site of thrombosis, and avoids another arterial puncture. Collateral circulation can be demonstrated by DSA. Prompt therapy

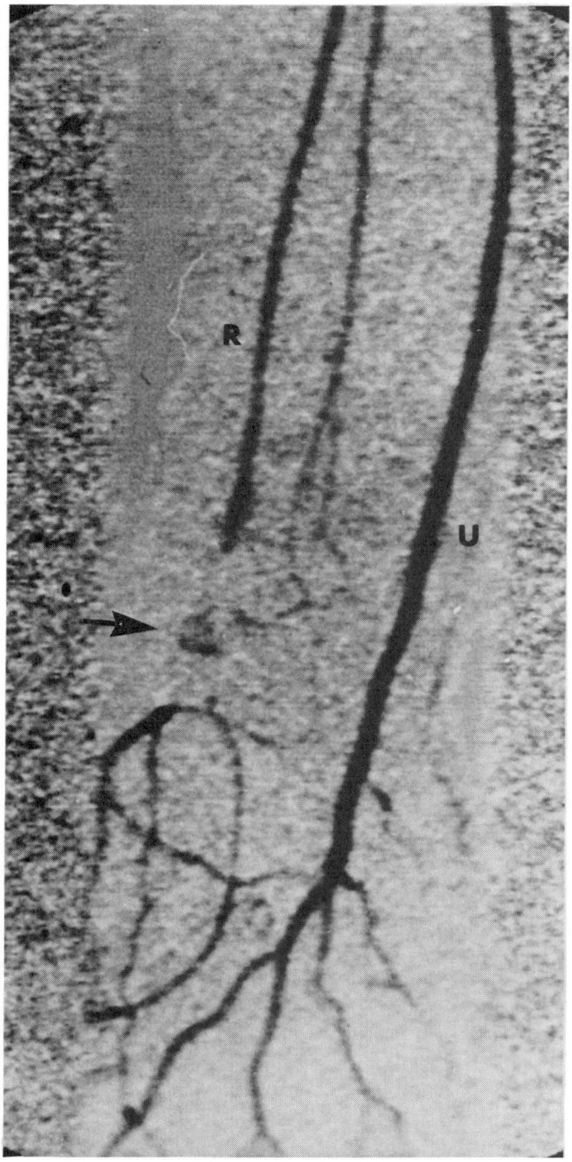

FIGURE 1. *Post-traumatic pseudoaneurysm (arrow) and occlusion of the radial artery (R) in a two and one-half-year-old boy. Note filling of palmar arcade via ulnar artery (U).*

is facilitated by precise diagnosis. Operative treatment of embolus has fairly good success in children older than two years, but surgery is technically difficult in those under two years and success of surgery is less certain.[40] Limb shortening can develop as a complication of untreated vascular occlusion.[41]

Dialysis graft problems can be evaluated by DSA without injection of the graft itself or of the feeding artery. The most common problem is stenosis of the arteriovenous shunt, usually on the venous side near the anastamosis. Such

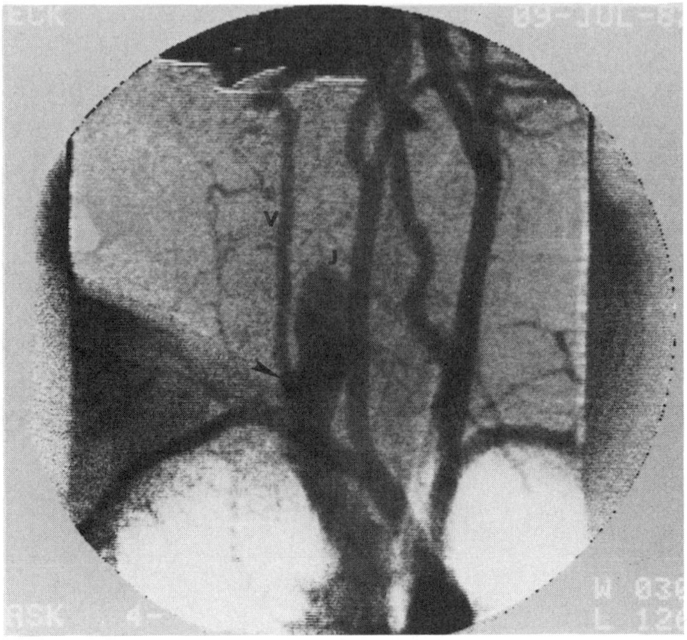

FIGURE 2. Post-traumatic fistula (arrow) between vertebral artery (V) and jugular vein (J) in a four-year-old boy. (Reprinted from Capitanio et al., Pediatr Clin N Am *32:1449–1460, 1985, with permission.)*

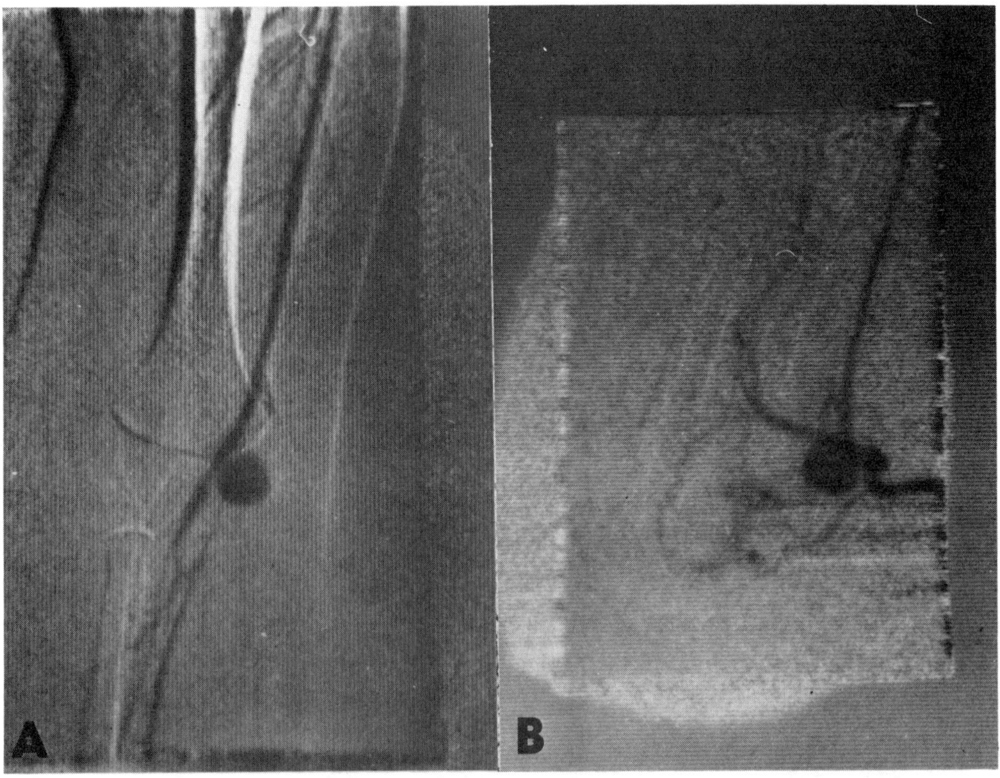

FIGURE 3. Post-traumatic pseudoaneurysm of brachial artery. ***A****: frontal view;* ***B****: lateral view. (Reprinted from Capitanio et al.,* Pediatr Clin N Am *32:1449–1460, 1985, with permission.)*

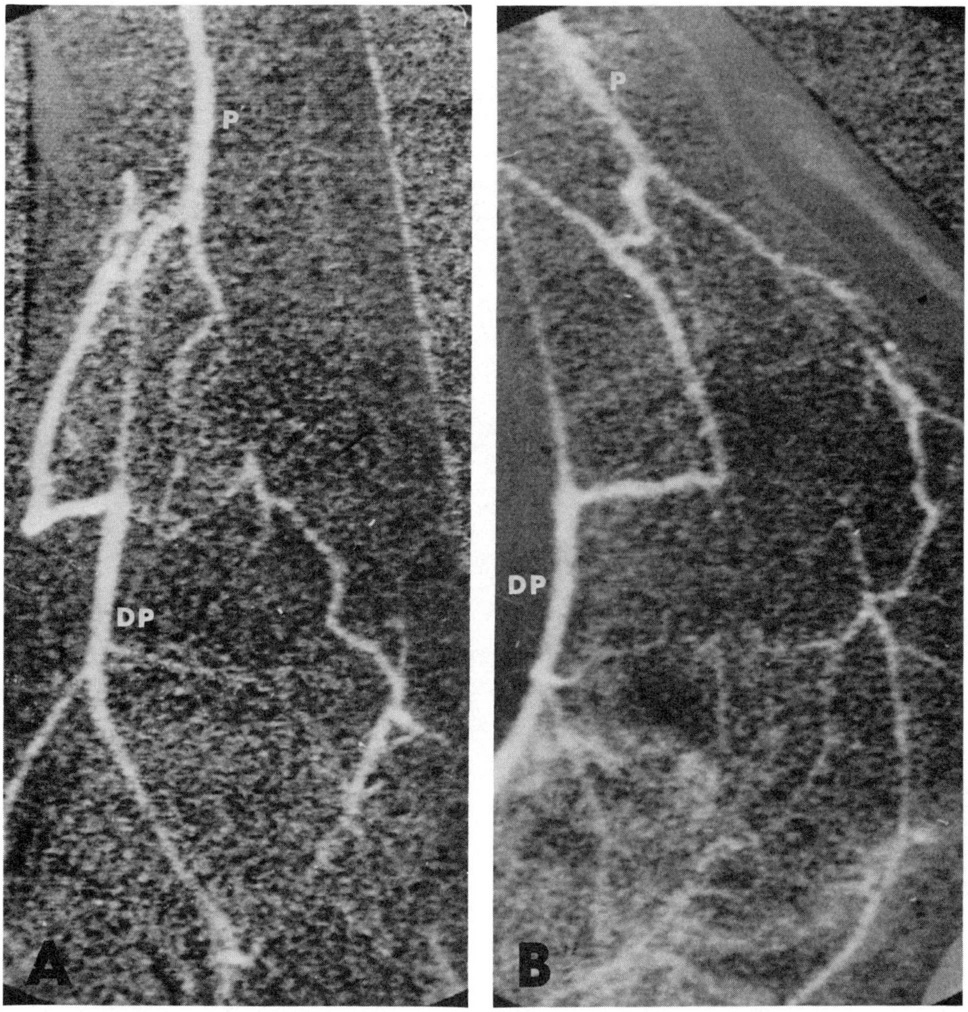

Figure 4. Obliteration of anterior tibial and posterior tibial arteries at the ankle following an electrical burn. ***A*** *frontal view;* ***B*** *lateral view. Note collateral vessel (arrow) from peroneal artery (P) supplying dorsalis pedis artery (DP).*

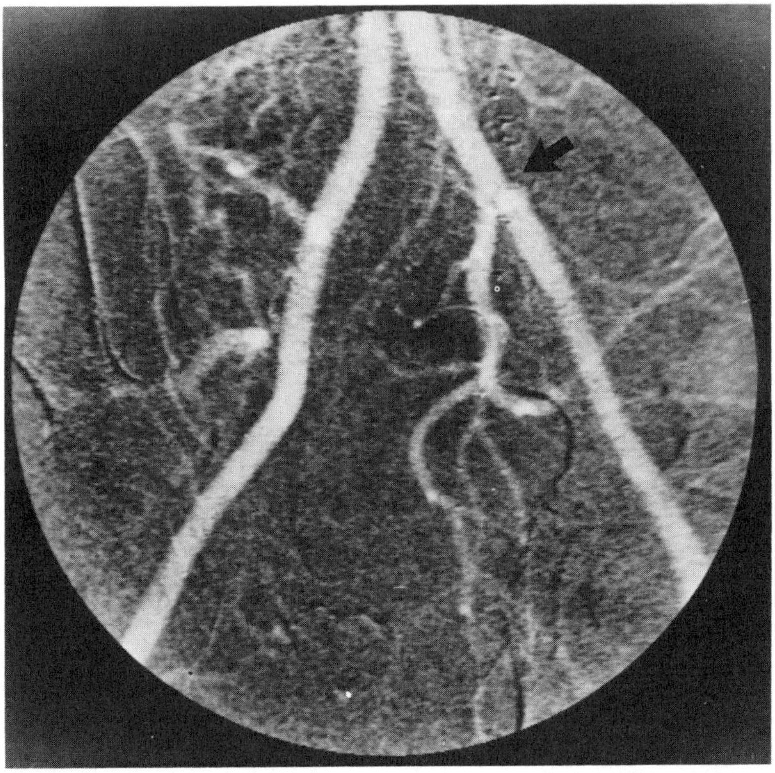

FIGURE 5. Iliac vessels after surgical transsection and reanastomosis of left external iliac artery just below bifurcation (arrow). The patient had developed claudication of the left leg. Right internal iliac artery diverted to supply previous renal allograft.

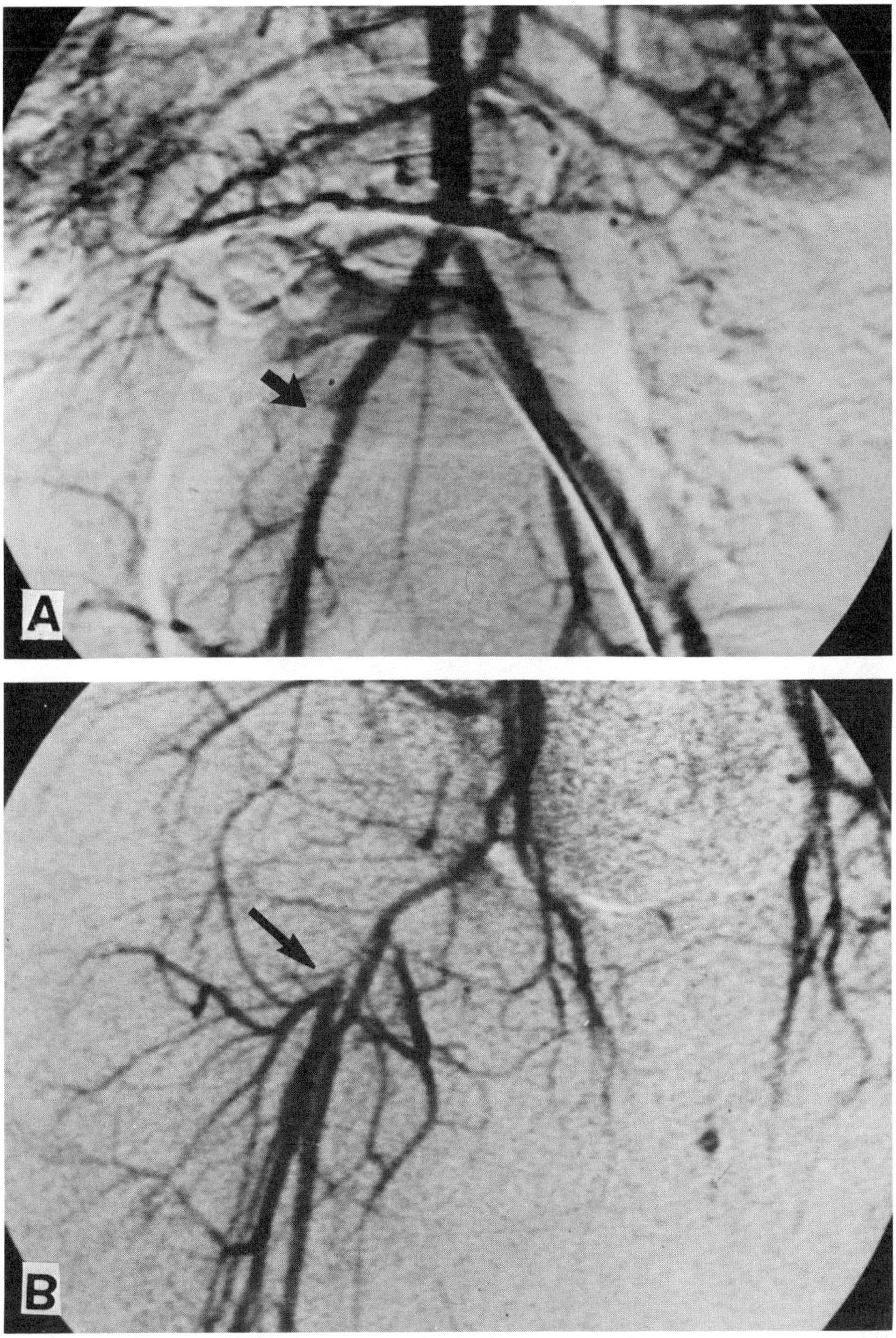

FIGURE 6. *A: Occlusion of right external iliac artery (arrow) following arterial catheterization. B: There is reconstitution of the femoral artery.*

shunts may also become occluded or form pseudoaneurysms at puncture sites.[42,43]

Vascular Malformations

Vascular malformations are congenital abnormalities of the blood channels and may be one of three types that are readily distinguishable by angiography. The first type, a direct arteriovenous connection, has large feeding arteries and early draining veins. The second type, a capillary malformation, may be seen only as a blush in the capillary phase (Fig. 7). In the third type, a venous malformation, the veins are enlarged and tortuous and there may be prolonged pooling of contrast in vascular spaces, but not much tissue staining.[33]

High flow with arteriovenous shunting may be present in an arteriovenous malformation.[44] These patients may have high output failure and cardiomegaly at presentation. Arteriovenous malformations of the extremities tend to be visible masses and angiography is not necessary for diagnosis, but is useful as a map for surgery or interventional occlusion. The lesions are usually well shown by DSA because they have enlarged vessels due to increased flow and shunting of blood (Fig. 8). Surgery is difficult as there are multiple feeding arteries and the malformations tend to recur if all the feeding arteries are not ligated. Embolization may be effective.[33]

Tumors

Angiography may be of value prior to surgery for bone and soft tissue tumors in demonstrating the relationship of a tumor to major vessels.[45] Information about the vasculature also helps in determining the surgical approach and in planning the need for amputation or extent of resection.[46] Both soft tissue and bone tumors can be evaluated by DSA[47,48] (Fig. 9). The vascularity as well as the extent and location of the tumor can be assessed by DSA. Tumor stains are better seen on DSA than on conventional angiography because of superior contrast enhancement of the digital system. In addition, the venous drainage of tumors is well seen. However, fine tumor vascularity may not be as well seen on DSA as on a conventional study. Although displacement of major vessels can be seen on DSA, encasement of vessels and subtle changes in caliber are not well shown.

Vasculitis

Vasculitis causing changes in large vessels can be demonstrated by DSA[10] (Figs. 10 and 11). Takayasu's arteritis is a vascular disorder that is considered to be autoimmune in nature. It causes fibrosis and thickening of the arterial wall of the aorta and its branches. In 75% of patients, one or both subclavian arteries are involved.[33,49] Arteriography shows diffuse or focal stenoses, sometimes accompanied by aneurysmal dilatation.[50] Collateral supply may develop around very severe areas of stricture.

Kawasaki's disease (mucocutaneous lymph node syndrome) is a disease of infants and young children characterized by fever, conjunctivitis, and adenopathy.[51] Aneurysms may appear in multiple organs. The etiology is unknown, but patients tend to respond to aspirin (Fig. 12).

Venography

Venography has been described using DSA techniques.[12] Thromboses, stenoses, and malformations of the veins may be shown using a venous peripheral injection of only 15% contrast.[17] The study is less painful than the conventional study and the subtraction technique eliminates bone overlap.

Intervention

Interventional procedures can be facilitated in children by use of DSA.[52] Availability of real-time fluoroscopic "road mapping" and the instant replay of video tape reduces catheter manipulation time and aids selective catheterization.[27] Since only small amounts of contrast medium are needed for a diagnostic study, both a diagnostic and therapeutic study can be carried out at the same sitting. DSA is used during angioplasty and immediately following the procedure to monitor the results. Follow-up studies in patients with recurrent symptoms after angioplasty are readily performed by DSA. DSA also may be used during embolization procedures to monitor the vascular occlusion following successive embolizations. Last but not least, DSA is useful in demonstrating the position of catheters placed for therapeutic infusion.

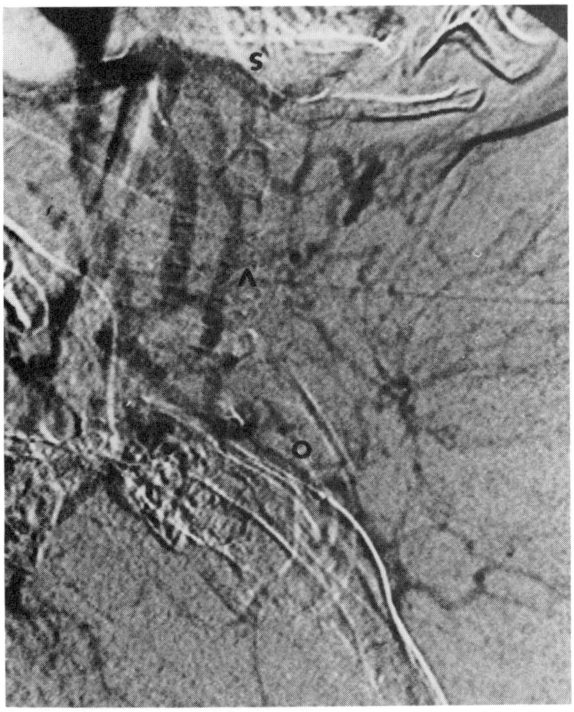

Figure 7. Large hemangioma of the neck with arterial branches from the subclavian artery (S), vertebral artery (V), and occipital artery (O).

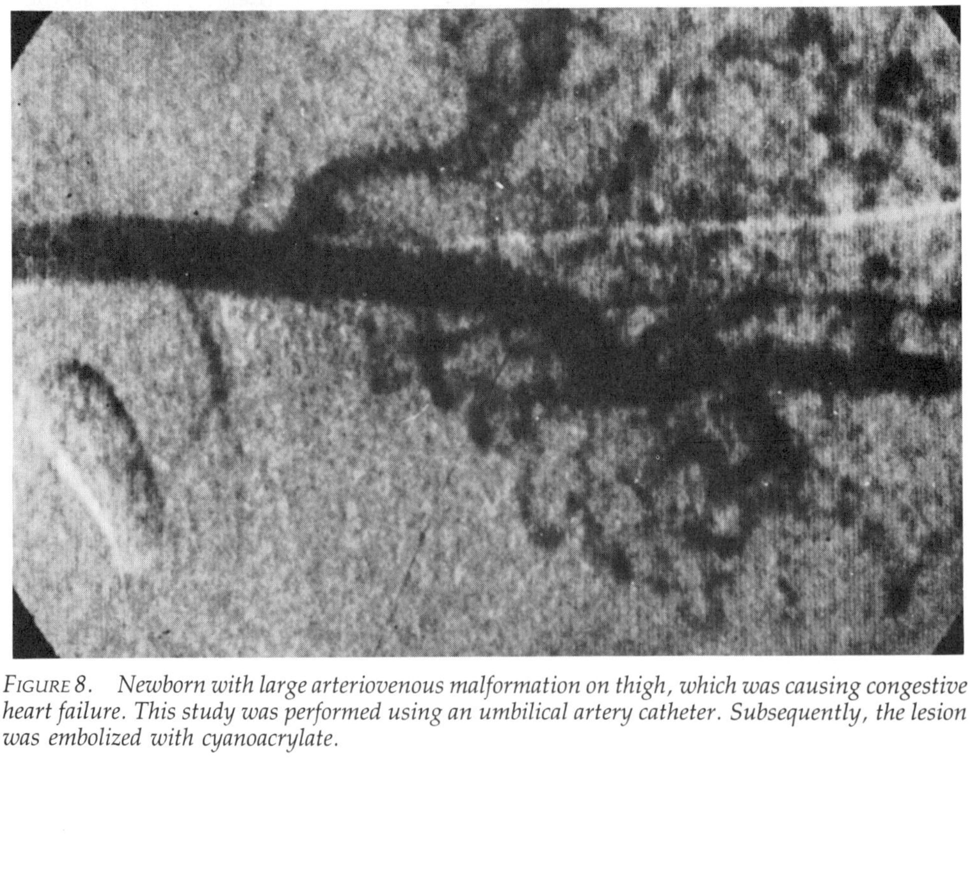

Figure 8. Newborn with large arteriovenous malformation on thigh, which was causing congestive heart failure. This study was performed using an umbilical artery catheter. Subsequently, the lesion was embolized with cyanoacrylate.

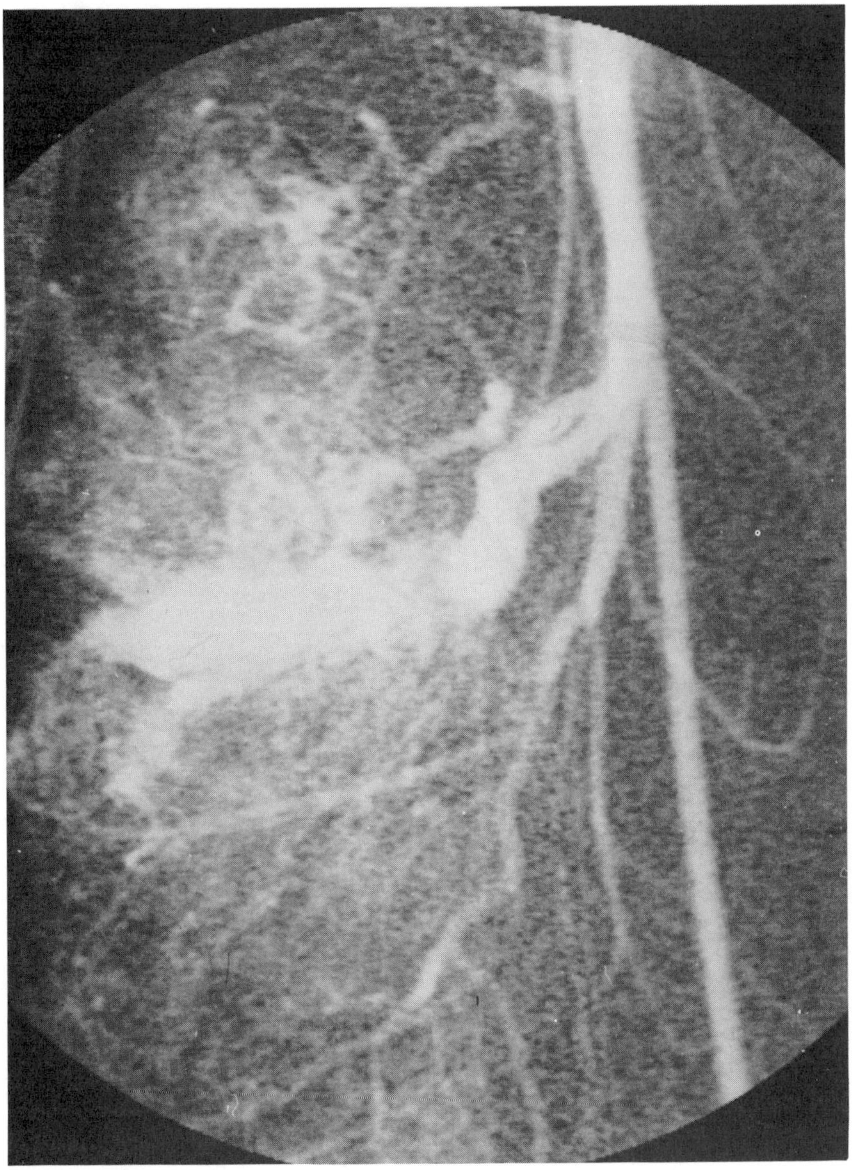

FIGURE 9. Lymphangioma of soft tissue of thigh.

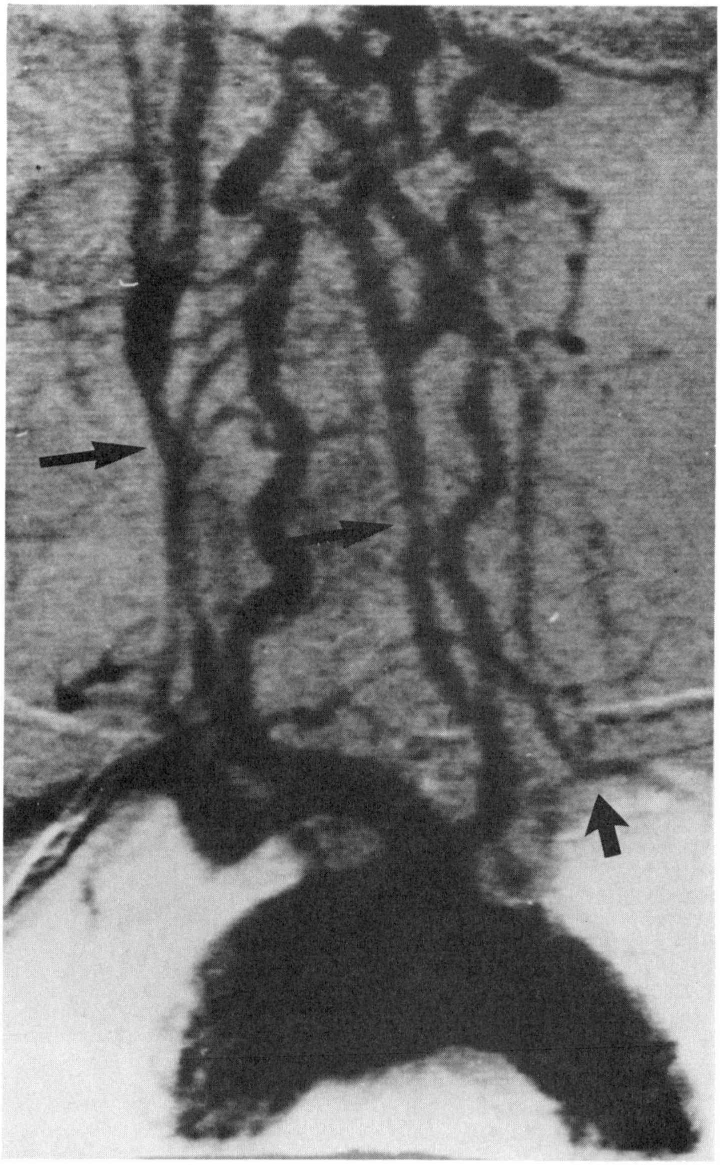

FIGURE 10. Takayasu's arteritis in four-year-old boy. Note marked narrowing of left subclavian artery (short arrow) and of both common carotid arteries (long arrows).

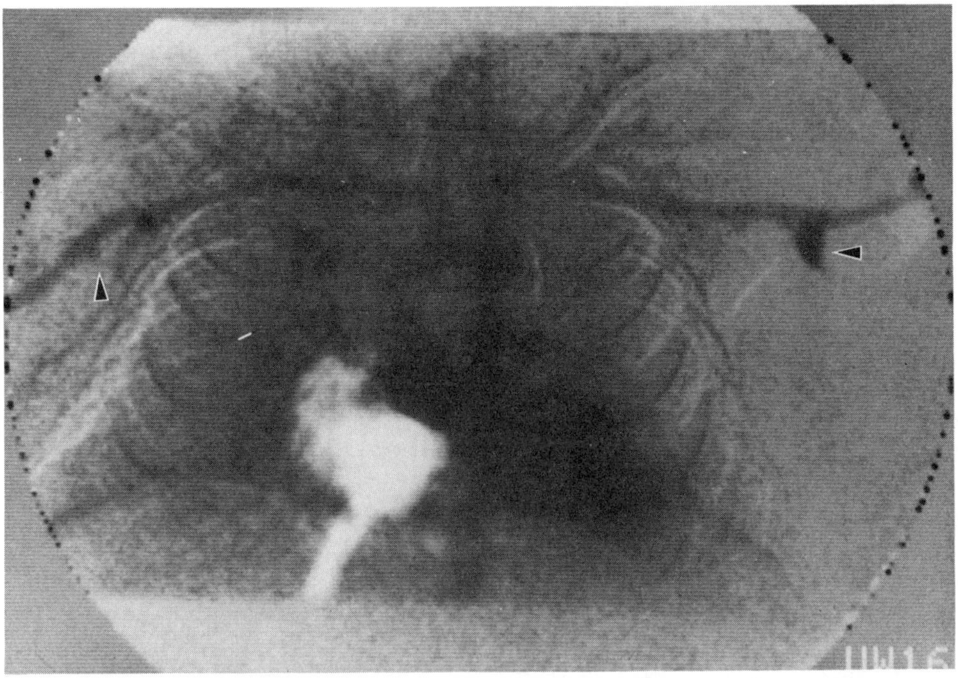

Figure 11. Polyarteritis nodosa in a four and one-half year-old boy. Note bilateral subclavian aneurysms (arrowheads). (Reprinted from Capitanio et al., Pediatr Clin N Am *32:1449–1460, 1985, with permission.)*

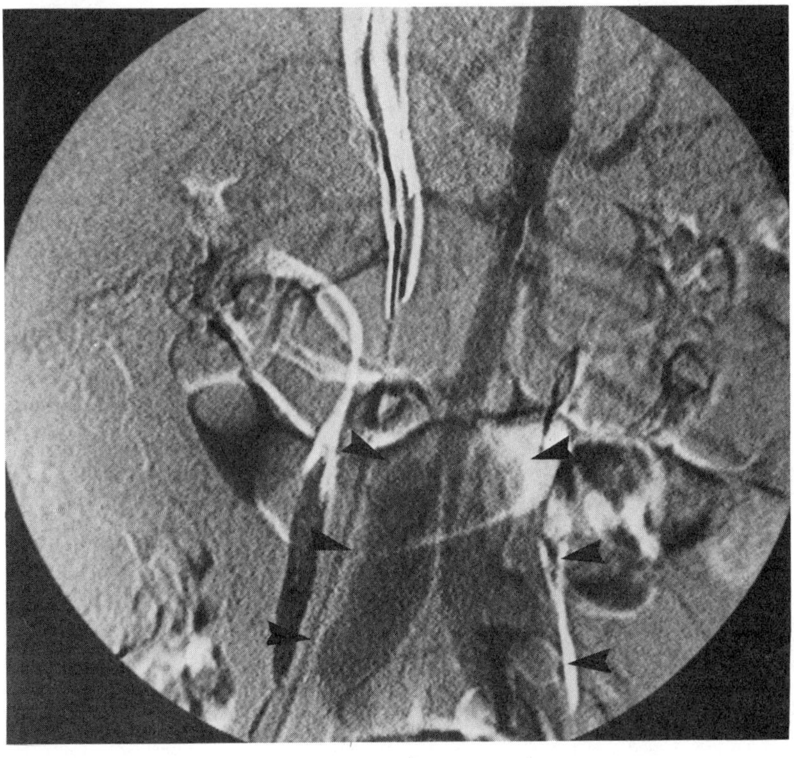

Figure 12. Bilateral fusiform aneurysms (arrows) of common iliac arteries in a three-month-old girl with Kawasaki's disease.

References

1. Crummy AB, Strother CM, Lieberman RP, et al: Digital video subtraction angiography for evaluation of peripheral vascular disease. *Radiology* 141:33–37, 1981.
2. Crummy AB, Strother CM, Sackett JF, et al: Computerized fluoroscopy: Digital subtraction for intravenous angiocardiography and arteriography. *AJR* 135:1131–1140, 1980.
3. Lewis BD, Enzmann DR, Guthaner DF, et al: A high frame-rate digital subtraction angiography imaging technique for evaluation of aortofemoral runoff. *Radiology* 151:789–790, 1984.
4. Ovitt TW, Christenson PC, Fisher HD III, et al: Intravenous angiography using digital video subtraction: X-ray imaging system. *AJR* 135:1141–1144, 1980.
5. Rosen RJ, Roven SJ, Taylor RF, et al: Evaluation of aorto-iliac occlusive disease by intravenous digital subtraction angiography. *Radiology* 148:7–8, 1983.
6. Turnipseed WD, Crummy AB, Strother C, et al: Computerized intravenous arteriography: A technique for visualizing the peripheral vascular system. *Surgery* 89:118–123, 1981.
7. Capitanio MA, Faerber EN, Gainey MA, et al: Digital subtraction angiography and its application in children. *Pediatr Clin North Am* 32:1449–1460, 1985.
8. Bunker SR, Cutaia FI, Fritz AL, et al: Femoral intraarterial digital angiography: An outpatient procedure. *AJR* 141:593–596, 1983.
9. Thompson JR, Schneider S, Ashwal S, et al: The choice of sedation for computed tomography in children: A prospective evaluation. *Radiology* 143:475–479, 1982.
10. Fitz CR, Harwood-Nash DC: Special procedure techniques in infants. *Radiol Clin North Am* 13:181–198, 1975.
11. Eskridge JM, Becker GJ, Rabe FE, et al: Digital vascular imaging: Practical aspects. *Radiology* 148:703–705, 1983.
12. Kadir S: Digital subtraction angiography (DSA). In: *Diagnostic angiography*. Philadelphia, PA: WB Saunders Co, 1986, pp. 103–123.
13. Rubin DL, Burbank FH, Bradley BR, et al: An experimental evaluation of central vs. peripheral injection for intravenous digital subtraction angiography (IV-DSA). *Invest Radiol* 19:30–35, 1984.
14. Saddekni S, Sos T, Sniderman KW, et al: Optimal injection technique for intravenous digital subtraction angiography. Animal and clinical studies of right atrial injection using small volumes (25 ml) at a high rate (35 ml/sec). *Radiology* 150:655–659, 1984.
15. Modic MT, Weinstein MA, Pavlicek W, et al: Intravenous digital subtraction angiography: Peripheral *versus* central injection of contrast material. *Radiology* 147:711–715, 1983.
16. Popky GL, Saluk PH, Griska LB, et al: Comparison of superior vena cava and antecubital vein as DSA injection site. *AJR* 143:317–319, 1984.
17. Amundson GM, Wesenberg RL, Mueller DL, et al: Pediatric digital subtraction angiography. *Radiology* 153:649–654, 1984.
18. Smith DC, Rold KD, Hewes RC, et al: The cephalic vein as an access route in intravenous digital subtraction angiography. *Br J Radiol* 58:670–672, 1985.
19. Burbank FH, Brody WR, Bradley BR: Effect of volume and rate of contrast medium injection on intravenous digital subtraction angiographic contrast medium curves. *J Am Coll Cardiol* 4:308–315, 1984.
20. Kaufman SL, Chang R, Kadir S, et al: Intraarterial digital subtraction angiography in diagnostic arteriography. *Radiology* 151:323–327, 1984.
21. Miller FJ, Mineau DE, Koehler RP, et al: Clinical intra-arterial digital subtraction imaging. Use of small volumes of iodinated contrast material or carbon dioxide. *Radiology* 148:273–278, 1983.
22. Gersten K, Pillari G, Greenspan B, et al: Crossed-leg technique for digital subtraction angiography. *AJR* 146:843–844, 1986.

23. Goodman PC, Jeffrey RB Jr, Brant-Zawadzki M: Digital subtraction angiography in extremity trauma. *Radiology* 153:61–64, 1984.
24. Pinto RS, Manuell M, Kricheff II: Complications of digital intravenous angiography: Experience in 2488 cervicocranial examinations. *AJR* 143:1295–1299, 1984.
25. Franken EA Jr, Girod DA, Sequeira FW, et al: Femoral artery spasm in children. Catheter size is the principal cause. *AJR* 138:295–298, 1982.
26. Crummy AB, Stieghorst MF, Turski PA, et al: Digital subtraction angiography: Current status and use of intra-arterial injection. *Radiology* 145:303–307, 1982.
27. Turski PA, Stieghorts MF, Strother CM, et al: Digital subtraction angiography "road map." *AJR* 139:1233–1234, 1982.
28. Passariello R, Rossi P, Simonetti G, et al: Digital subtraction angiography for examination of vessels of the leg: Use of a 40 cm image intensifier. *Radiology* 149:669–674, 1983.
29. Chakravarty M: Utilization of angiography in trauma. *Radiol Clin North Am* 24:383–396, 1986.
30. Love L, Braun T: Arteriography of peripheral vascular trauma. *AJR* 102:431–440, 1968.
31. McDonald EJ Jr, Goodman PC, Winestock DP: The clinical indications for arteriography in trauma to the extremity. *Radiology* 116:45–47, 1975.
32. Smith PL, Lim WN, Ferris EJ, et al: Emergency arteriography in extremity trauma: Assessment of indications. *AJR* 137:803–807, 1981.
33. Zelch MG, Geisinger MA: Arteriography of the extremities. In Taveras JM, Ferrucci JT (Eds): *Radiology, Diagnosis–Imaging–Intervention* Vol 2. Philadelphia, PA: J B Lippincott Co, 1986, pp. 1–16.
34. Lang EK: The role of arteriography in trauma. *Radiol Clin N Am* 14:353–370, 1976.
35. Hofammann KE III, Moneim MS, Omer GE, et al: Brachial artery disruption following closed posterior elbow dislocation in a child—Assessment with intravenous digital angiography. A case report with review of the literature. *Clin Orthop* 184:145–149, 1984.
36. Holland BA, Jeffrey RB, Brant-Zawadzki M: Intravenous digital subtraction angiography in the demonstration of femoral pseudoaneurysms. *AJR* 141:607–608, 1983.
37. Fabian TC, Reiter CB, Gold RE, et al: Digital venous angiography. A prospective evaluation in peripheral arterial trauma. *Ann Surg* 199:710–716, 1984.
38. Perry MO: Iatrogenic injuries of arteries in infants. *Surg Gynecol Obstet* 157:415–418, 1983.
39. Picus D, Totty WG: Iatrogenic femoral arteriovenous fistulae: Evaluation by digital vascular imaging. *AJR* 142:567–570, 1984.
40. Smith C, Green RM: Pediatric vascular injuries. *Surgery* 90:20–31, 1981.
41. Mortensson W: Effects of percutaneous femoral artery catheterization on leg growth in infants and children. *Acta Radiol Diagn* 21:297–302, Fasc 2B, 1980.
42. Boomsma JHB, Beukhof JR, Geerlings W, et al: *Diagn Imaging Clin Med* 53:243, 1984.
43. Butler P: Intravenous digital subtraction angiography. *Br J Hosp Med* 35:30–36, 1986.
44. Burrows PE, Mulliken JB, Fellows KE, et al: Childhood hemangiomas and vascular malformations: Angiographic differentiation. *AJR* 141:483–488, 1983.
45. Hudson TM, Enneking WF, Hawkins IF Jr: The value of angiography in planning surgical treatment of bone tumors. *Radiology* 138:283–292, 1981.
46. Paushter DM, Borkowski GP, Buonocore E, et al: Digital subtraction angiography for preoperative evaluation of extremity tumors. *AJR* 141:129–133, 1983.
47. Takahashi M, Koga Y, Bussaka H, et al: The value of digital subtraction angiography in peripheral vascular diseases. *Br J Radiol* 57:123–32, 1984.
48. Lee KR, Cox GG, Price HI, et al: Intraarterial digital subtraction arteriographic evaluation of extremity tumors: Comparison with conventional arteriography. *Radiology* 158:255–258, 1986.
49. Mishima Y: Arterial insufficiency of the upper extremity with special reference to Takayasu's arteritis and Buerger's disease. *J Cardiovasc Surg* 23:105–108, 1982.

50. Arey JB: Vascular diseases. In: *Cardiovascular Pathology in Infants and Children*. Philadelphia, PA: WB Saunders Co, 1984, pp. 352–355.
51. Kawasaki T, Kosaki F, Okawa S, et al: A new infantile acute febrile mucocutaneous lymph node syndrome (MLNS) prevailing in Japan. *Pediatrics* 54:271–276, 1974.
52. Katzen BT: Peripheral, abdominal, and interventional applications of DSA. *Radiol Clin North Am* 23:227–241, 1985.

Chapter 9

Future Applications and Trends in Digital Imaging

H. THEODORE HARCKE

Introduction

Technology has now successfully produced high-quality digital images with all of the modalities of our specialty except for the most basic and most commonly requested—the plain film. Consider the major techniques available for producing images: x-ray attenuation, ultrasound interaction, radiographic tracer emission, and magnetic resonance (MR). The latter three processes have digital images ready to be integrated into a system designed to archive, retrieve, and transfer information. In the category of x-ray attenuation, successful imaging has been accomplished in two special areas: computed tomography (CT) and subtraction angiography. The fundamental and most frequently performed x-ray examination, the plain film, is now in the process of being digitized. Therefore, we are certain that in the future there will be total digital imaging; the real question is: how fast will we progress to this end?

There is no doubt that the key to total digital imaging lies with the development of acceptable nonangiographic radiographic imaging systems. An equally challenging task is the integration of all modalities in their digital form. A number of factors will determine the rate at which nonangiographic digital imaging can progress and the totality of medical imaging can become an integrated, purely digital process. We tend to concentrate the most on technical issues such as speed of acquisition, resolution, and storage, but the problems of implementation are equally formidable. Even when we have the technology to produce digital plain films that would give acceptable resolution in comparison to current film screen images, the cost of converting to digital technology will undoubtedly prohibit rapid change. There are also the human factors. Hendee has pointed out two fundamental problems confronting the practice of radiology today: (1) the selection of studies (triaging) of a patient in radiology and

Digital Subtraction Imaging in Infants and Children, edited by Eric N. Faerber. Mount Kisco, New York: Futura Publishing Company, Inc., © 1989.

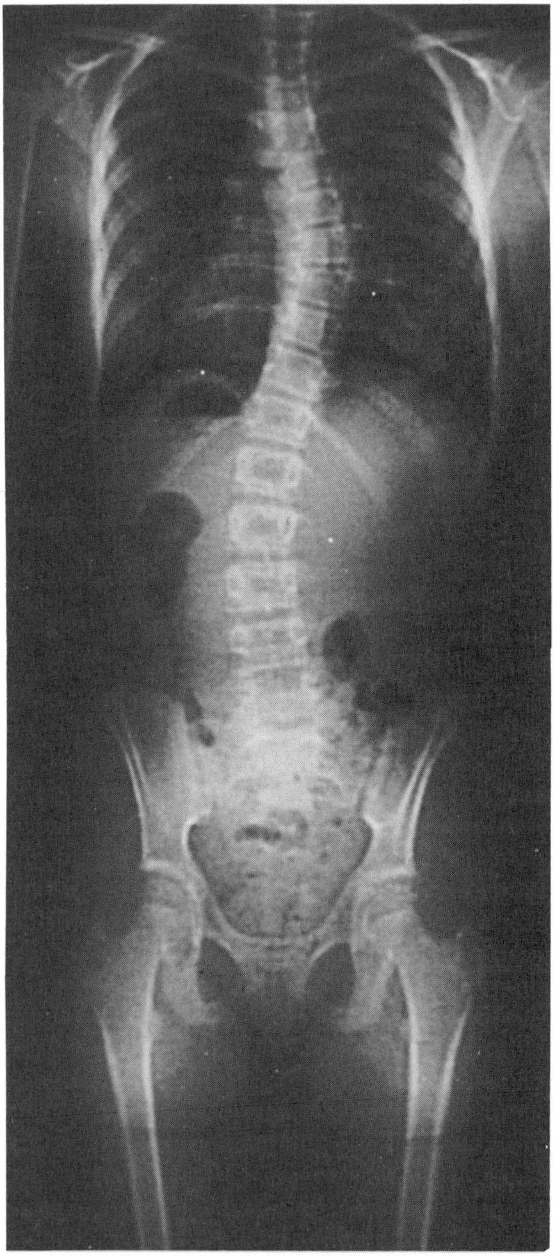

FIGURE 1. Digital images of the spine give acceptable resolution for the follow-up of scoliosis. With this technique, radiation exposure is very low, approximately 2 mR per image.

(2) provision of a consensus radiologic diagnosis following the patient's evaluation by multiple modalities.[1] Although integrated digital radiology systems provide a means to deal more effectively with these two aspects of radiologic practice, they require a change from the style of radiology practice that has evolved in the past two decades. There are threatening elements to the linking of modalities into a central system because this counters the present-day trend of subspecialization by modality. On the other hand, integrated digital systems offer a viable solution to the organization of the radiology department on an organ system basis, a practice that is common at university centers.

At our institution, the Alfred I. duPont Institute, a high percentage of the plain film studies involve the skeleton. Two thirds of these constitute follow-up examinations, such as a posteroanterior film of the spine to evaluate an adolescent with scoliosis or a standing film of the lower extremities to assess limb deformity in a child. We made an early commitment to nonangiographic digital radiography because our somewhat unique needs were met by current technology and because the system we selected provided acceptable digital images at a substantial reduction in radiation exposure (Fig. 1).[2] In this final chapter, as I speculate about nonangiographic digital imaging and the integration of all modalities, it will be tempered with the experience gained using one of the first "plain film" digital systems in a clinical pediatric radiology environment. In implementing and operating our system, we have come face to face with many of the basic issues and questions that relate to the future.

Present Issues

It is fruitless to try to discuss in great detail current nonangiographic digital technology. Even as this is being written, information is changing and equipment manufacturers are proceeding in several directions. A general overview of nonangiographic digital technology, however, brings out most of the issues that touch upon the integration of all modalities into an electronic/digital picture archiving and communications system (PACS). It is convenient to look at technologic issues from four aspects: image acquisition and formatting, display and manipulation, image archiving, and the network.

Image Acquisition and Formatting

There are two strategies that result in the production of a digital radiograph. The true digital radiographic system involves a process in which the x-ray beam interacts with an x-ray-sensitive detector other than a conventional film screen system. The interaction produces a signal that must be converted to digital form and processed by computer in order to become visible. Although there are systems that convert a processed radiograph to a digital form, I do not consider these to meet the definition of a true digital radiographic system. This is not to say that such systems will not play a role in the radiology department of the future. At the Alfred I. duPont Institute, we currently have all of our plain films and most special studies recorded on film and face the problem of integrating the old study and the new as true digital radiographic images are produced.

There are a number of possible configurations for true digital systems, and these make use of a variety of x-ray source and detector combinations.[3] The CT localization film, for example, is a digital plain radiograph with which most are familiar. The x-ray source is a fan beam sector that strikes a closed circular array of detectors. As the patient moves slowly through the stationary source/detector configuration, a patient image is generated by a series of projections from a pulse source.

As an alternative, a scan system can move the source and detector while the patient remains stationary. Both fan beam and pencil beam sources are being utilized. The latter approach, the collimation of the source to a pencil beam configuration that scans the patient line by line, is the basis for our digital system, the American Science and Engineering (Cambridge, MA) Model 1500 (Fig. 2). The source and solid-state detector move in synchrony, and the field is scanned by the system. Depending on the size of the patient and the field to be studied, the process involves 5 to 12 sec. It is imperative that the patient not move during this time interval.

A number of manufacturers have chosen to work with analog recording of the full x-ray beam on a sensitive plate. This technique possesses a time advantage over the scanning beam system in that exposures are of the speed used

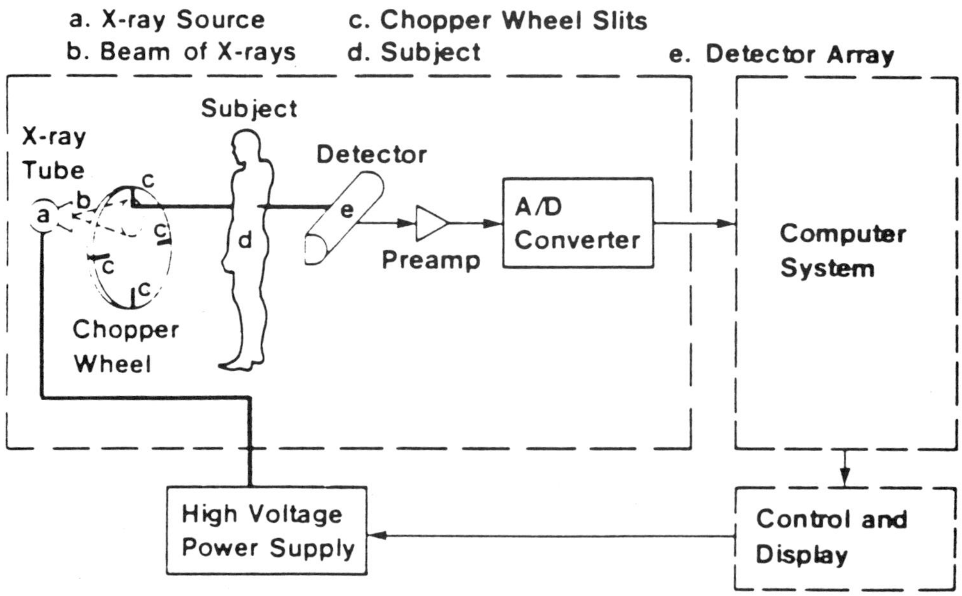

FIGURE 2. Schematic representation of the American Science and Engineering digital radiographic system. The pencil beam source (a, b, and c) and detector (e) move together to scan the stationary patient (d). (Diagram reproduced courtesy of AS&E, Inc., Cambridge, MA.)

with conventional film/screen radiography even when pediatric studies are being performed. The plate containing the image is scanned by a laser, which activates the image. The activated image is read and converted to a digital format.[4] This type of process has an important economic advantage that accounts for its popularity: existing x-ray generators are used in conversion of existing radiographic rooms to digital technology without totally abandoning equipment in place. In addition, when malformation occurs in the digital system, a conventional film/screen study can be substituted and the room is not totally useless.

Display and Image Manipulation

The advantages in display and processing that digital images have over analog images are clear. Typically, the digitized patient image is converted to an analog signal for display on a video monitor. The immediate availability of the image for viewing is superior to the conventional film process in which there is a delay between the image acquisition and the availability of the image. Incorrect positioning or the need for an additional view can be established before the patient has left the procedure room. Also, by viewing each image in sequence, it is possible to eliminate views that are now done routinely and may be unnecessary when a lesion or abnormality is clearly identified on a first or second image. Presently, there are some limitations to this concept of immediate access. When multiple images are acquired, such as in CT, the console is often locked out for viewing during the acquisition of the next image and, therefore, is not available for viewing or processing. Systems utilizing reusable stimulable phosphor plates require processing of the plate before the image is displayed.

Like CT, digital systems assign gray-scale intensity values to ranges of pixel values with the viewer interactively able to control window width (range of values from black to white) and window level (the center of the range of values to be displayed). This important and primary advantage of a digital image allows the viewer to see multiple images from a single acquired image. All are familiar with the ability to manipulate contrast so that optimal visualization of bone and soft tissue can be made from a single CT slice. This same technique applied to digital chest radiographs has enhanced visualization of lung abnormalities and constitutes the fundamental reason for the interest in nonangiographic digital technology.[5] When this technique is applied to extremity examinations, one can obtain the equivalent of a bone radiograph and soft-tissue radiograph from the same exposure. It should also emphasized that the ability to manipulate a digital image eliminates the need for retakes due to improper exposure. Although I concur with this, it is important to remember that retakes necessitated by motion and incorrect positioning still occur.

Improvements in the contrast ratio of objects to be detected are also achieved by manipulation of digital images. At the Alfred I. duPont Institute, in fact, we found that our radiologists preferred an enhanced digital image to the basic digital image when performing measurements of spinal curvature (Fig. 3). Initially, our system performed contrast enhancement as a separate step after a

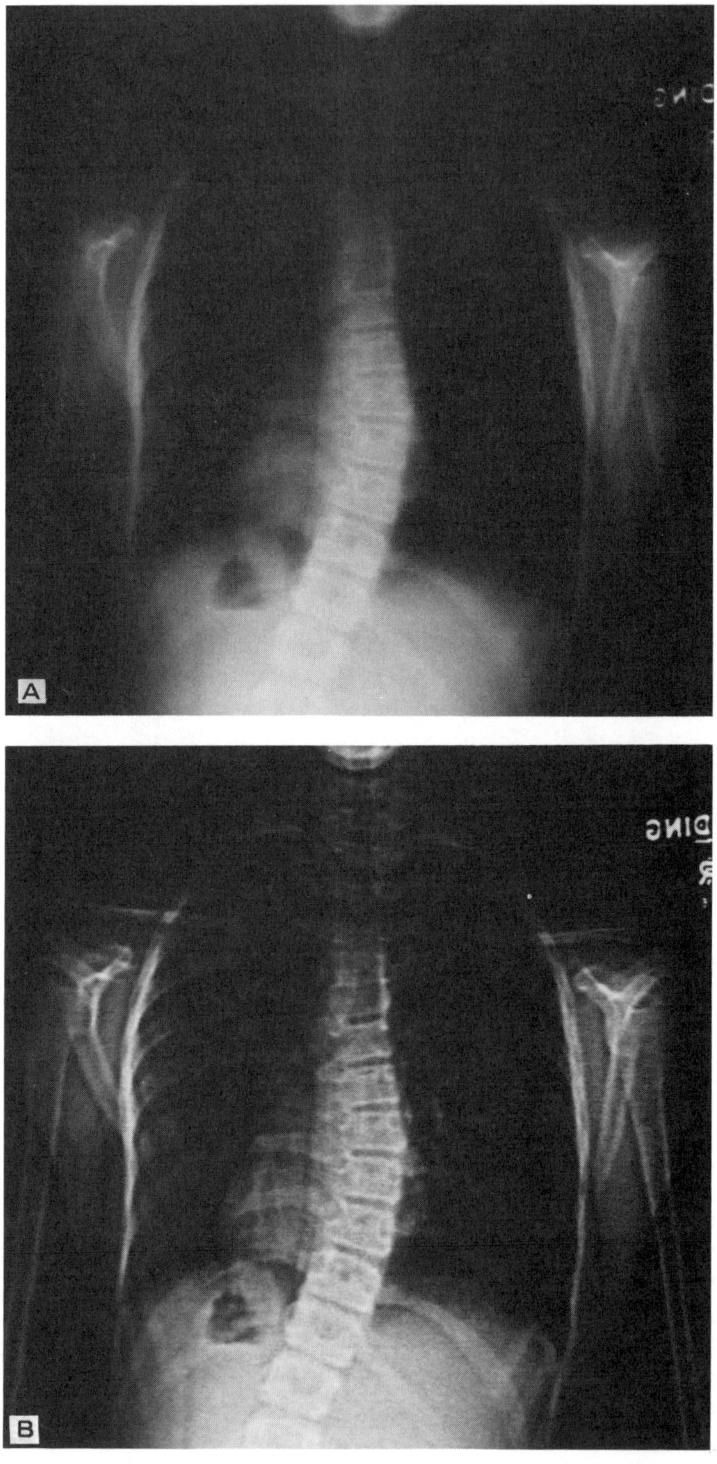

Figure 3. *A digital radiograph is many images in one. Computer manipulation permits enhancement of image contrast.* ***A****: Unprocessed digital radiograph of the thorax.* ***B****: After contrast enhancement, the detail of the dorsal spine is clearer and measurement of scoliosis was judged to be easier.*

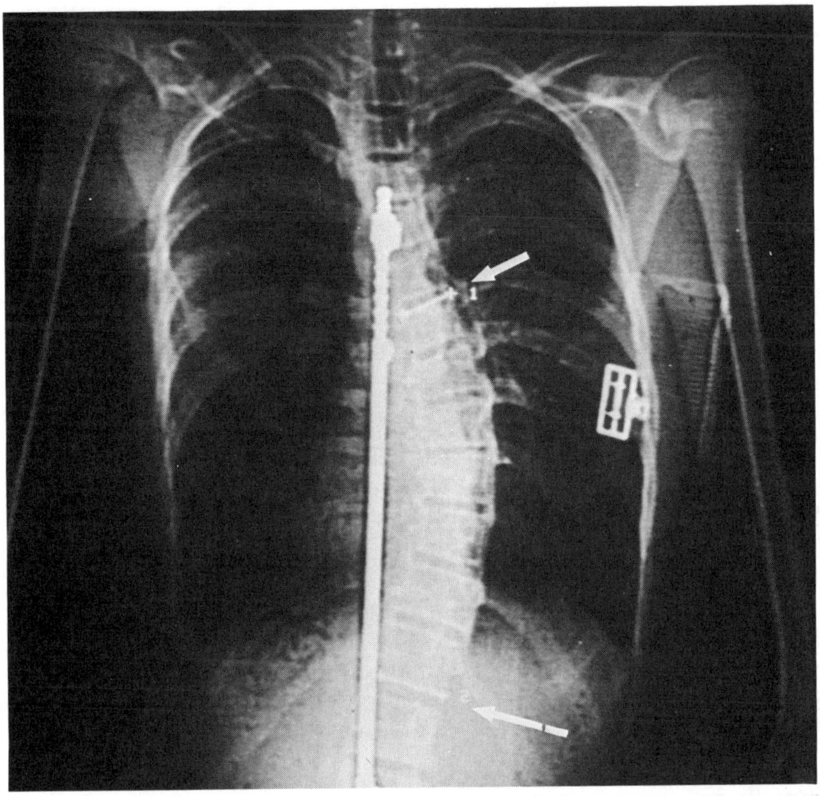

FIGURE 4. *Angles of spinal curvature can be measured directly on digital images using computer software. After the viewer places the cursors to identify the points of reference (arrows) the angle measurement is calculated and displayed on the monitor (not shown).*

complete image was acquired. This step, which took between 2 and 3 min, prolonged the time of each patient's examination and adversely affected patient throughput in our unit. The problem was readily solved, however, through the installation of a board that allowed initiation of processing as the image was being acquired. We now have an enhanced image available for viewing 11 to 14 sec after completion of the acquisition. This experience is mentioned because it illustrates two points: (1) the initial design of a digital system is not always the most efficient from the standpoint of clinical use, and (2) the capabilities exist to modify digital systems so that they can maintain their inherent advantages and still maximize clinical utility.

Digital systems possess a capability for measurement that is lacking on conventional film images. Measurement consists not only of relative tissue attenuation in regions of interest but also of linear and volumetric measurements. These already have been incorporated into CT, nuclear medicine, and ultrasound software and are available on plain film digital systems as well. At our institution, our orthopedic applications are particularly concerned with angular measurement (degree of spinal curvature in scoliosis) (Fig. 4) and linear measurement (bone-length discrepancy). When we began to use digital technology, we performed controlled studies comparing measurement of spinal curvature and leg-length discrepancy done by digital technique with conventional film technique.

Spinal curvature calculated on our digital unit measured an average of 2.6 degrees higher than that calculated on conventional radiographs. This was determined to be due to a variation in x-ray beam geometry in our digital system.[6] We also discovered that measurement of digital images by different observers was more variable than angular measurement on conventional radiographs. This is attributed to the miniaturization encountered with the display of the digital image. A slight variation in landmark selection results in a potentially greater angular variation than on larger "life-size" conventional images.

Measurement of leg-length discrepancy on our digital system (Fig. 5) was compared with that on conventional orthoroentgenograms. In phantom studies, we found that because of the divergent x-ray beam, the conventional three-exposure orthoroentgenogram was actually less accurate than the digital system when measuring patients with significant leg-length inequalities. Our patient studies confirm the overall accuracy of digital radiography and the feasibility of performing measurements with the patients standing as opposed to the supine positioning for the conventional orthoroentgenogram.[7]

Our work with comparative measurements emphasized the importance of performing controlled studies of comparative measurement when introducing digital techniques. There will be subtle differences in measurements with different units, and the human interaction with the miniaturized image on the video terminal introduces factors that must be considered when making comparisons with measurements from conventional analog films.

The immediate availability of a digital image for viewing not only is an advantage at the site of acquisition and processing within the imaging department but also affords clinicians the opportunity to view a study before the patient returns to the office or clinic. The placement of terminals for display and manipulation is an important consideration in digital imaging. The cost of interactive terminals is considerably greater than display-only terminals, and each institution will have to assess the need for a viewer to manipulate data or merely view data. The advantage of seeing a variety of images from one set of data is lost when the viewer cannot interact. From a practical point, however, a substantial number of terminals throughout the hospital will likely be for viewing only. This limits the viewer at that terminal from experiencing the advantage of the extended dynamic range contained in the electronic image. We placed a remote interactive terminal in the orthopedic clinic of our hospital so that clinicians could have the same ability as the radiologists to change the level and window and perform other measurement functions. We have encountered several problems that have resulted in underutilization. Maintaining a basic level of training for personnel proved impossible. Staff physicians did not want to take the time to learn the system, resident physicians were constantly changing, and other clinic personnel such as orthopedic assistants and nurses were rotated. We also found that in a busy clinic, the presence of only one monitor caused a

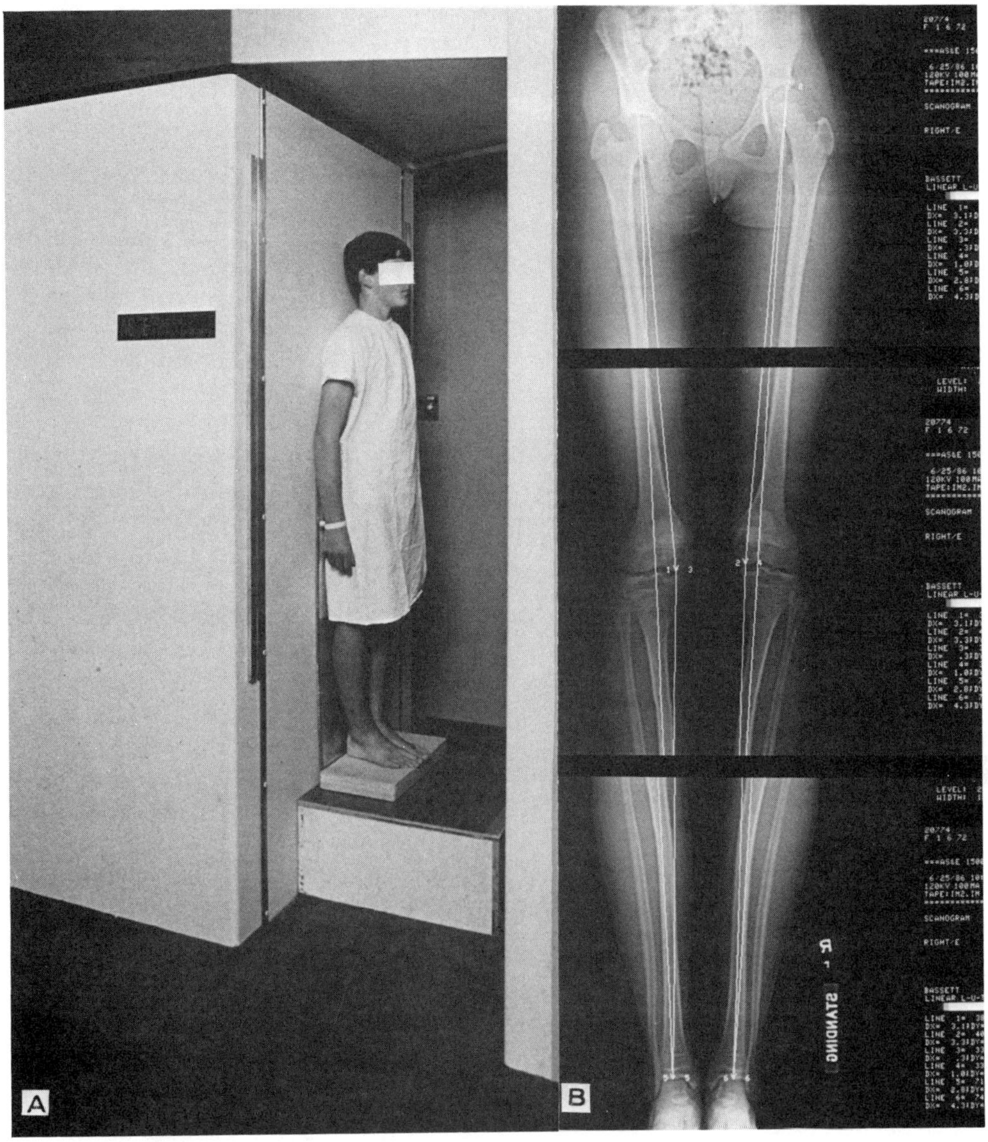

*FIGURE 5. **A:** Digital measurement of leg length. The patient stands in the gantry and is scanned by a moving x-ray source. **B:** Digital measurement of leg length. Digital displays show three segments of the study annotated for calculation of bone length. By convention, the delta y (Dy) component represents actual limb-length difference.*

back-up when several residents wanted to use the system for measuring and viewing at the same time. None of the problems we observed with the interactive terminal are unsolvable, but they illustrate a general point: introduction of new technology that forces a change in the style of clinical practice will meet resistance to acceptance.

Image Archiving

A major concern of those using digitally formatted imaging systems is the storage and retrieval of data. Current problems in our film file rooms are lamentable: the tedious practices of logging studies into film jackets, signing jackets in and out from the department for conferences and clinics, and the search for missing films and/or missing folders. We look to digital systems as a means of salvation. In theory, although the storage and retrieval of digital information should solve many of our problems, there is a new set of problems inherent in the "digital file room." The sheer amount of digitally formatted data that will be acquired for display and archiving is overwhelming. Already, busy departments with existing digital modalities can generate as much as 900 megabytes of data per working day.[8] At present, most departments not only store the digital data but also continue to produce multiformat film recordings of the studies that are maintained in separate or centralized film libraries with other patient imaging studies. Faced with the requirements to maintain patient files for a minimum of five years for adults and up to age 21 for pediatric records, maintenance of dual sets of data is likely to occur for some time in the future. The prospect of digitizing existing film records, although feasible, not only is costly but also poses a problem for the digital archives. The present popular use of magnetic tape is recognized as inadequate. The logistics and efforts required to retrieve and re-enter data stored on magnetic tape exceed those required for handling current film records. It is a very intricate and time-consuming process, and the only advantage is the saving of space.

It is generally recognized that requirements for the archiving and retrieval of data depend on the type of patient and on the time elapsed from completion of the study. For inpatients, there is an initial period of high demand for access to the patient's imaging data. This is fostered by the need for review by the staff member rendering the report, the desire of other staff members to view a study for comparison with one done by another modality, and the demand for review by referring physicians and house staff. This initial period of high demand should end within 24 to 48 hours of the time of acquisition. A period of moderate demand for the study generally follows the period in which a patient is hospitalized. There are times when a study will need to be compared with subsequent imaging studies obtained during hospitalization, and key portions of a study will be required for review during rounds and conferences. After discharge, there is a low demand for access to the patient's imaging data. Data may need to be reviewed during an outpatient visit and for comparison with follow-up studies. In the initial high-demand period, it is desirable to retrieve data in terms of seconds; during the period of moderate demand, it is also preferable to have rapid access to data. During the low-demand period, personnel maintaining files should be able to retrieve data and transfer it to a rapid access status within minutes.

Like other hospitals, we currently archive our present digital imaging modalities on discs to meet the requirements of the high- and moderate-demand periods. It is then customary to retain the data on magnetic tape during the low-demand period. Our digital radiographic unit uses this general scheme with some modification. Because the majority of our digital radiographic studies are performed on outpatients, there is no real demand for the data several hours after acquisition of the study. A further factor in reducing the demand for the digital data in our hospital is our practice of recording selected images on film. In order to minimize the amount of data stored and recorded, we transfer to magnetic tape only the raw images and do not permanently record any of the enhanced images or images showing measurements. Conversely, the images multiformatted and recorded on film are limited to an enhanced spine image (Fig. 3B) or the leg-length images showing the measurement data (Fig. 5B). In this way, we have minimized archiving in both respects, on tape and on hard copy. To review the patient's previous digital study on a monitor, we must transfer the information from tape to disc, repeat the image-enhancement process, and redo the measurement. Clearly, there is a need for new technology that will meet the demand for storage of vast quantities of digital data and permit accessing with varying amounts of speed.

Our experience with digital radiographic studies of an orthopedic nature pointed out the existence of a human factor in the use of digital images. Our orthopedic colleagues, accustomed to viewing analog film images on viewboxes, expressed difficulty in looking at miniaturized images of the spine displayed on the video monitor or as a multiformatted image on film. The miniaturization factor made it difficult for them to judge the patient balance and degrees of rotation and to visualize the severity of the curve, all of which they felt very comfortable doing on conventional-sized film. They also expressed difficulty in comparing the digital image with the previous study when that study was on conventional film (14 × 36 in). We suspect that this is a transient phenomenon and that, with time, our colleagues will find no more difficulty in viewing the digital radiographic images than they do in looking at the minified images produced by the other digital modalities which we use.

Networks

The task of tying together the acquisition, display, and storage of different digital imaging modalities is being addressed independently by large departments and commercially by a large number of companies. Terms such as "image management systems" and "integrated diagnostics" have become common. In 1981, Duerinckx coined the acronym PACS, which stands for "picture archiving and communication system."[9] This term has survived in large part because of a series of technical conferences jointly sponsored by professional societies such as the Society for Optical Engineering (SPIE) and the Institute of Electrical and Electronic Engineers (IEEE). The problem of joining together different types of imaging equipment built by multiple manufacturers through computer systems made by other manufacturers introduces the obvious need for intermodality and intercompany compatibility. This is being done through the American College of Radiology–National Electrical Manufacturers Association (ACR-NEMA) Digital Imaging and Communications Standard. Such cooperative efforts are required for progress.

At every level, there are complexities that challenge the integration of the separate modalities. Digital images from nuclear medicine, CT, and ultrasound can be displayed on 512 × 10 bit matrices, but subtraction angiography and current digital radiographs need 1,024 × 1,024 × 12 bit matrices. There is work indicating that in order to achieve acceptable spacial resolution, digital radiographs will require 2,048 × 2,048 × 12 bit images.[10] Even the physical means by which one can connect a local network within a department requires technical decisions. A twisted wire, coaxial cables, fiberoptics, and combinations of these offer choices that are influenced by the type of data to be transmitted, distance, maintenance, ability to upgrade, and, certainly, cost of installation.

Our digital radiographic system embodies the simplest form of network. We have linked the acquisition and processing terminal to a physician's console, a remote viewing and processing terminal, and a storage device (Fig. 6). From such a simple network, we have learned that planning and implementation involve a number of choices. Location of any single component of the system has advantages and disadvantages that need to be weighed. Often, structural and space limitations will prevent desired configurations.

When one begins to add additional components to the network, the configuration of the links that connect the components, in particular the computer elements, is known as network topology. Most work to date has been done on local area networks that link together components within a radiology department. These typical networks involve the linkage of image acquisition and formatting devices with a station for image display and manipulation. Stations for display and manipulation should be capable of transferring data to and from

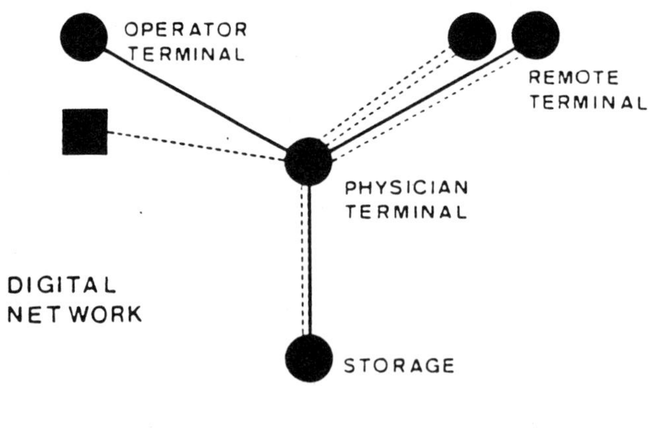

FIGURE 6. Simple digital radiographic network. The operator and physician terminals are within the radiology department, and the remote terminal is in the orthopaedic clinic. Solid lines show present operation. Dotted lines indicate future expansion.

any acquisition area in the system and of displaying studies from any diagnostic imaging modality. It is, in fact, preferable to be able to produce an interactive display where different modalities can be viewed on the same video terminal. The whole process of network communication is predicated upon a set of priorities. Communicating efficiently within the system is not an easy task, particularly when a system is designed with no centralized communications controller.

Another aspect of a network extends beyond the local area of the department and involves peripheral locations such as remote offices, other hospitals, or even the physician's home. This is coupled with the desirability of connecting the department's system with the management and information system of the hospital as a whole.

The Future

We see the future in the present. Already, some departments estimate that almost twenty-five percent of their total examinations are digitally formatted.[8] The growth of magnetic resonance imaging (MRI) will bring a new modality that is already in digital form. The thrust of technology within the field of medical imaging is toward the concept of the all-digital department with integration of the modalities. Coupled with this plan for integration are the current investigations in the field of teleradiology and other transmission systems that can link imaging facilities miles apart.

In the immediate future, larger institutions will work hand in hand with industry to establish evaluation sites for large multimodality PACS. Initially, these will deal with present day digital modalities of CT, MRI, subtraction angiography, nuclear medicine, and ultrasound. As prototypical plain digital radiographic systems become available, these will be integrated. At another level, single subsystems will be linked. These local PAC systems are already found in areas such as nuclear medicine, in which a series of gamma cameras are linked to a central system for display and processing.

What we are likely to see, therefore, is a series of phased integrations. Beginning with integration within a single modality such as nuclear medicine, a next step would be to integrate nuclear medicine with CT and MR images. Although we already envision this type of process, methods for implementation, particularly with respect to storage and archiving, are less clear. The ability of present storage systems to handle large quantities of digital data and satisfy the demand for the initial period of high utilization, subsequent moderate utilization, and eventual low-demand, long-term storage has not been established. The technology of long-term archiving is changing. Although we have relied on magnetic discs and tapes, it is likely that future technology will involve optical and solid-state storage devices, and these will bring acceptable solutions. There will still be the problem of maintaining dual systems, because film will continue to play a role for some time to come. In a department with mixed analog and digital modalities, film continues to offer a convenient means for recording the formatted digital information. It will be some time before hospitals are willing to commit the resources to convert to totally digital systems. The cost of placing terminals throughout an institution as well as the conversion of existing film records to digital format will ensure that dual systems are present for some time to come.

As the technology becomes available to integrate imaging within radiology, its acceptance will not be automatic. The ability of the radiologist to adjust to the digital era will be a factor. In the past, radiology has followed a trend toward subspecialization by modality. Fellowships were and still are offered in CT, ultrasound, nuclear medicine, and magnetic resonance imaging. As long as education by modality continues, there is likely to be some reluctance for the radiologist to allow his or her territory to be invaded by others at the stroke of a keyboard. On the other hand, if the subspecialization of radiology shifts to an organ system approach such as we have seen with neuroradiology, the integrated imaging systems should be welcomed with enthusiasm. It would be possible for the chest radiologist, for example, to have the patient's plain film, CT scan and lung scan displayed on a console with ultimate ease. The specialty of imaging itself, then, can influence the future of digital imaging as well as being influenced by it.

Whether the radiologist of the future practices as an organ system expert or a modality expert, it is likely that there will be a trend toward consensus reading. By this it is meant that a consultation incorporating a series of imaging studies will be rendered by the radiology group. It will consider the information provided by each of the independent modalities with its inherent strength and weakness. The consultation will integrate the information for the referring physician and provide him or her with the most likely diagnosis (or diagnoses) based on the total imaging data. There is no doubt that in accomplishing this, the radiologist will be receiving the information digitally, viewing and processing the information at a video terminal, and even transmitting the consensus report digitally to its destination. Just as the radiologist of the past was found in front of a viewbox, so the radiologist of the future will be found in front of a computer terminal.

References

1. Hendee WR: Digital Radiography in International Symposium, The Impact of New Imaging Technology on Health Care, Research, and Teaching: 2. What is to be expected in the future? *AJR* 142:190; 1984.
2. Kushner DC, Cleveland RH, Herman TE, et al: Radiation dose reduction in the evaluation of scoliosis: An application of digital radiography. *Radiology* 161:175–181, 1986.
3. Vizy, KN: An overview of digital radiography systems. *Cardiovasc Intervent Radiol* 6:1, 1983.
4. Sonoda M, Takano M, Miyahara J, et al: Computed radiology utilizing scanner laser stimulated luminescence. *Radiology* 148:833–838, 1983.
5. Fraser RG, Eamann B, Barnes GT: Digital radiography of the chest: Clinical experience with a prototype model. *Radiology* 148:1–5, 1983.
6. Harcke HT, Mandell GA, Lee MS, et al: Evaluating scoliosis with digital radiographic techniques. (Abstract) *AJR* 145:875, 1985.

7. Altongy JF, Harcke HT, Bowen JR: Measurement of leg-length inequalities by MicroDose[R] digital radiographs. *J Pediatr Orthop* (in press).
8. Cox GG, Templeton AW, Dwyer SJ: Digital image management: Networking, display, and archiving. *Radiol Clin N Am* 24:37–54, 1986.
9. Duerinckx AJ (Ed): Proceedings of the 1st International Conference and Workshop on Picture/Archiving and Communication Systems (PACS) for Medical Applications, Newport Beach, California, January 18–21, 1982.
10. Seeley GW, Newell JD II: The use of psychophysical principles in the design of a total digital radiology department. *Radiol Clin N Am* 23:341–348, 1985.

Appendix

Design and Staffing Considerations in a Pediatric Digital Angiographic Suite

SUZANNE E. BRICKLEY

Digital subtraction equipment is now commonly found in most major hospitals. Because of its widespread applications, it fulfills the needs of many different departments, such as radiology, cardiology, neurology, neurosurgery, and surgery. In the pediatric setting it may be possible to combine the digital procedures performed by all departments by creating a facility such as the one at St. Christopher's Hospital for Children.

The addition of digital subtraction imaging equipment to the cardiac catheterization laboratory with biplane facilities enables flexibility to perform a digital subtraction study instead of, or in addition to, conventional angiography during a cardiac catheterization procedure. It is thus not necessary to decide beforehand which procedure will be performed.

Most digital subtraction angiography (DSA) studies referred from the radiology department are outpatient elective procedures that can be performed along with the daily inpatient cardiac DSA studies. This enables better utilization of the total facility and staff. Standard cardiac angiographic procedures and DSA are complimentary, not competitive modalities. The ever increasing applications of DSA have made it part of the daily routine in angiography departments.

At St. Christopher's Hospital for Children, the cardiac catheterization technical staff provide on call service for both cardiac and radiologic emergency procedures. Personnel (technologists, nurses) should be certified in advanced life support techniques and familiar with operation of emergency (code) equipment.

I. Digital Equipment

A. Hardware. All equipment listed below is used for routine DSA

Digital Subtraction Imaging in Infants and Children, edited by Eric N. Faerber. Mount Kisco, New York: Futura Publishing Company, Inc., © 1989.

studies, with the exception of the analytical processing unit (APU). The applications of the APU is discussed in Chapter 4.

1. Systems desk containing:
    - 2 CRT
    - keyboard
    - joy stick
    - short-term storage for Analog/Capricorn disc
    - long-term storage (digitally stored) Winchester disc
    - 525-line T.V. chain with fluoroscopy
    - analytical processing unit

B. Software

1. Analytical Programs. The three analytical programs listed below are the most frequently used in the post processing of data.
    - interpolative zoom: increases magnification of region of interest
    - pixel shift: mask offset
    - contour enhancement: adds dimension
2. Additional Analytical Programs
    - ejection fractions and regional wall motions: cardiac contractility measurements
    - calibration and subsequent length measurement: used primarily to assist in angioplasty and valvuloplasty

II. Life Support Equipment. All rooms in which DSA is performed should have full life support systems

A. Oxygen administration and suction capability

B. Oxygen and air outlets: respirator hook up

C. Defibrillator
- pediatric and adult paddles
- cardioversion capability

D. Physiological monitor
- electrocardiogram: all patients
- arterial pressure: required during arterial catheterization
- skin temperature monitoring: neonate and infant

E. Crash cart with standard resuscitation capabilities

F. Patient temperature regulation equipment
- heat blanket: aquamatic
- radiant warmer ceiling lamps
- neonatal thinsulate bunting

III. Instruments. Custom disposable digital subtraction angiography kit

A. Skin prep equipment
- Povidine iodine swabsticks (3)
- fenestrated drape with adhesive
- 6 absorbent towels
- 2 towels with adhesive
- 72″ sheet

B. Physician gown with towel
C. Patient drapes
D. Skin infiltration
  - 10-cc disp. Luer-Lok syringe
  - 18 ga × 1½″ aspirating needle
  - 25 ga × ⅝″ infiltration needle
E. Percutaneous needles
  - 21 ga or 19 ga Potts Cournand needle
  - 21 ga or 19 ga clear hub arterial needle
  - 21 ga butterfly needle
F. Instruments
  - #11 scalpel with handle
  - 1 guide wire bowl
  - 1 medicine glass
  - 2 towel clips
G. Disposable supplies
  - 3-way stopcock
  - 20″ high pressure contrast injector tubing
  - 4 × 4 gauze sponges (50)
  - 12″ adhesive tape (2)
H. Fluoro covers (2)
  - image intensifier cover
  - radiation protection shield
I. PVP (Povidine iodine) ointment
J. IV flush
  - IV tubing
  - 250-mL D5W .025 saline with 500 units heparin

IV. Catheters and Accessories
  A. Power Injector with 1000 PSI Capability
  B. Disposable 100 cc Syringes—Clear
  C. Catheter Introduction
    - *Cardiac*: Percutaneous Sheath Introducer Sets
      Intravenous and Intra-arterial Insertion
        4F to 7F
    - *Radiologic*: Seldinger Technique
      Intravenous
        4F dilator tapered to .032
      Intra-arterial
        3F dilator tapered to .021
        4F dilator tapered to .032
        5F dilator tapered to .035 or .038
  D. Catheters
    - *Cardiac*:
      Intravenous
        NIH, Berman, high-flow NIH

Intraarterial
as above, plus high-flow pigtail

- *Radiologic*:
  Intravenous
  4F high-flow straight flush
  IVC injection, cerebral, renal, and peripheral applications
  Intraarterial
  selective vessel catheters, as indicated (3F–5F)

INDEX